— THE —
HIBERNATION DIET

— THE —
HIBERNATION DIET
IT WORKS WHILE YOU SLEEP

Mike and Stuart McInnes
with
Maggie Stanfield

SOUVENIR PRESS

Typeset by FiSH Books, Enfield, Middx
Printed in Great Britain by Bookmarque

Contents

Get the Buzz – A New Way of Thinking and Eating   1

What's it all about?   1

Not the biology I was taught!   2

So what do I need to do?   3

How the Hibernation Diet Works   4

How does this great miracle work?   7

'Tired all the time'   12

Night nonsense   13

Morning sickness   15

Slow Wave Sleep   16

Heroic resistance exercise   19

Healthy Eating   21

Body-friendly foods   22

The food quiz   22

The Hibernation Diet food circle   24

Golden rules   26

Go shopping   26

A word about cooking   28

The Hibernation honey-eating plan   29

Get the Hibernation Habit: Eating Outlines   31
  Prime time   31
  In-between time   33
  Lunch time   33
  Blue time one   34
  Blue time two   35
  Dinner time   36
  Bed time   37
  Hibernation honey drinks   38

Join the Heroic Resistance Movement   43
  What resistance work isn't   43
  What resistance work is   43
  The home resistance movement   46
  The resistance routine   47
  Advice for gym members   52
  Benefits for everyone   53

The Birds and the Bees   55
  The hungry brain   57

How to Be a Hibernation Diet Expert   59
  Hunger: where and what is it?   59
  Fat: where and what is it?   64
  Hibernation Diet metabolic personalities   67
  Test yourself   70

How to Achieve a Sense of Wellbeing   73
  Food and stress   73
  Exercise and stress   76
  Depression and Weight   79

Tired All the Time   85
  Weighing it all up   88

So What *Am* I Eating?   95
   Fats   95
   Proteins   96
   Carbohydrates   98
   Food for thought   99
   Female food   102
   Food and children   103
   Give the dog a bone   104
   A life on the ocean wave   105
   Immune food   105
   The junk food jungle diet   106
   Food and forgetfulness   106
   Gut food feeling   108

Life, Love and Leisure   109
   Hanna's story   110
   Everything is in order   113
   Kirsten's story   114

APPENDIX   117
Supplements and the Hibernation Diet   117
   To Supplement or not to supplement   117
   Nutrition in health   118
   Obesity   119
   Diabetes   122
   The immune function   123
   Depression   126
   Irritable Bowel Syndrome   129
   The thinking function   130
   Cardiovascular health and high blood pressure 131

Glossary of Terms   133
Bibliography   148
About the Authors   151

Get the Buzz – A New Way of Thinking and Eating

Lose weight while you sleep? Madness? Impossible? Not at all. What's more, you'll discover energy resources you never knew you had. You'll wake up feeling refreshed and ready for a demanding day ahead, and your whole body will benefit.

Your skin will improve its tone and texture. Your hair, your nails, your internal organs, your mood will all reap the benefits of the Hibernation Diet.

You will feel better at work, in your leisure time – even your sex life will be improved.

WHAT'S IT ALL ABOUT?

Heard the buzzword, TATT? Tired All The Time. Doctors say it's the most common complaint they hear. Worn out, exhausted, no energy, flaked out, dog tired, just want to sleep. Why?

We aren't working with our bodies. We're working against them all the time, and nature doesn't like that so it fights back to our detriment.

The Hibernation Diet is entirely different from all other fad, low-calorie and food-excluding diets. Yes, you can sleep, and lose weight all at the same time. Miraculous? Not at all. This is no gimmick, no quack diet. What's different about the Hibernation Diet is that it's based on our biology. It works for us, not against us.

NOT THE BIOLOGY I WAS TAUGHT!

If you grew up calorie counting and being told never to eat at night, our ideas may sound strange to you. The Hibernation Diet is about recruiting your own natural recovery system for weight control. So stop thinking that you have to fight your body every inch of the way to get a healthy weight. You don't have to. You need to learn how to make it work for you. It's yours. Your body is your partner, not your enemy. It's an amazing piece of high precision human engineering that even the most advanced technologies cannot begin to match.

The science isn't complicated. It's just been ignored. Maybe it was too obvious to notice, because the Hibernation Diet is really common sense. You'll find out more as you read on, but here are the main ingredients:

- Your brain is a greedy monster that demands constant energy
- Your brain cannot store energy
- The energy it uses comes, first off, from your liver
- Your liver can only store a small amount of energy at a time – about 75 grams
- During the night, your body needs energy to build new cells for your bones, your skin, your muscles and all your vital functions
- It's your recovery gland, known as the pituitary, master of the recovery hormone production, that sends out the message, while you're asleep, to do all this reconditioning
- Working through your liver, your body spends at

least four hours a night doing all this calorie-demanding maintenance work
- And where do you get the calories from? Answer: your fat stores – nowhere else

The Hibernation Diet is about making your body work for you. Think loads of energy, of not tiring out, of being on top of whatever you want to do. A dream? Not at all. The Hibernation Diet will see you feeling as busy as a bee and that's no coincidence. It's those honey bees that hold the key.

SO WHAT DO I NEED TO DO?

- We want you to **listen** to your own body
- We want you to **understand** just a little biology
- We want you to **discover** the difference between glucose and fructose
- We want you to **find out** why the honey bees have the answer
- We want you to **feel better** than you've ever felt in your life
- We want you to **lose weight** sensibly and easily
- We want you to **sleep it off!**

How the Hibernation Diet Works

If you woke up tomorrow morning and dreamed you'd got thinner during the night, you'd think, 'Oh yeah, great. If only!' But that's just what you could be doing with the Hibernation Diet.

With it, you can turn this dream into your reality. We'll show you how to use the first four hours of sleep, called Slow Wave Sleep, to do just that. Those first hours are when you sleep most deeply and when your overnight repair systems are at their busiest.

You can persuade your body to burn up fat while you sleep so that you wake up not only slimmer but feeling fitter and healthier. It's human-scale hedgehog hibernation. Miraculous? Yes, and it remains one of the best-kept secrets in human biology. If you get this right, make sure that your body knows the luxury of Slow Wave Sleep and how to use it to your advantage, you stand to:

- **See all your recovery mechanisms working better**
- **Speed up your fat burning metabolism**
- **Cut back stress hormones**
- **Sleep better**

As your stress levels fall your overall mood and mindset will be far better. You'll feel healthier and happier.

If all this still seems too good to be true, we'll make you this promise:

The Hibernation Diet will lead the way forward to a new and better life.

Ask yourself a few questions:

Do you wake regularly during the night?
Do you suffer from restless sleep?
Do you suffer from night sweats?
Do you experience acid reflux during the night?
Do you have to go to the bathroom during the night?
Do you wake up exhausted in the morning?
Do you feel nauseous in the early morning?
Do you have a dry throat in the morning?
Do you suffer from night cramps?
Do you feel weak in the early morning?

If you've answered 'yes' to any of these questions, then it could be because you haven't fuelled up your liver for the night, so you've produced a tidal wave of stress hormones while you slept.

As a result, you've not enjoyed the benefits you're entitled to from that Slow Wave Sleep.

Those factors mean you'll wake up feeling dehydrated, your recovery – or pituitary – gland won't have been able to get on with its repairs, and you'll have lost bone mass. Your muscles will be weaker, your blood pressure higher than it needs to be, and you may well feel nauseous so that you can't eat a good breakfast.

Instead of burning fat, repairing your muscles and bones and inhibiting stress hormone production, you're actually in a negative energy balance. Your brain has been working off degraded muscle and bone throughout the night. Far from feeling refreshed from your night's sleep, you might as well have stayed up all night and run a marathon.

In the Hibernation Diet we will show you how to maximise your fat-burning potential during the miracle of Slow Wave Sleep, how to use the real and nature-intended benefit of the night fast (as animals do in hibernation) and how to reduce production of the dangerous hormones which cause so much distress and ill health.

NOCTURNAL MATHS

This is maths for dummies, so don't worry. We used a calculator.

We'll assume you sleep for 8 hours a night. An average female of, say, 5 foot 6 inches and 9½ stone is probably burning about 60 calories an hour. During your Slow Wave Sleep, you are burning 240. With three resistance routines a week (which will be explained later) you will increase that to 600 calories each night in that four-hour period. During lighter sleep, you will still burn 50 per cent more calories than otherwise, so you'll bring the 240 to 360, a total of 960 a night: 6,720 in a week, so doubling your fat metabolism.

Compare that with one full hour of pounding your heart out on the treadmill. That will result in 1,000 calories used. But 500 of these come from carbohydrates, including converted muscle, 200 come from muscle stores so have no effect on body fat at all. A miserable 300 come from body fat stores, equivalent to 33 fat grams of loss.

Fat is 9 calories to 1 gram, so 6,720 ÷ 9 = 746 fat grams a week, or three quarters of a kilo of pure fat loss – much more efficient than other diets which lose muscle and water, giving a false picture of weight loss. To get that loss from running on the treadmill, you'd have to do 20 one-hour sessions a week.

And that's all coming from your fat stores to rebuild all your organs, bone, tissue and muscle.

It's a lot more effective than pounding it out on a treadmill where you're burning up calories out of your vital muscle mass.

HOW DOES THIS GREAT MIRACLE WORK?

There are five pillars:

- **Honey**
- **Healthy eating**
- **Hibernation**
- **Hormones**
- **Heroic resistance**

We don't want to blind you with science, so we'll strip these crucial elements down to straightforward 'bites'.

Honey

Honey is one of the oldest foods known to man. The ancient Greek mathematician, philosopher and thinker, Pythagoras, who was born about 580 BC, affirmed the therapeutic properties of honey in his writings. He and his disciples used it as a central component in their strict but very healthy diet made up of vegetables, almonds and other nuts, figs and honey. The ancient Egyptians were well aware of it too and archaeological surveys have shown the high regard in which honey was held. For our purpose, honey is important because its molecules are half glucose and half fructose. That matters because, for our brain to access vital fuel from our liver, fructose has to free it up first. It's the only way the brain can take it in.

Healthy eating

What we eat shows. White bread, pizza, burgers, chips, pints of beer and cider, crisps and sugary tea or coffee add up to fat people. Wholemeal and granary bread, fresh fruit and vegetables, loads of water and fresh, lean meat, fish and organic poultry without additives add up to slim, fit, healthy and full of vitality. Okay, it's not quite that simple, but it's not too difficult either.

Hibernation

Lots of animals feed themselves up over the summer, sleep through the winter and come out slim and famished. Why? Obviously they live off stored fat. What we're forgetting is that, though we don't hibernate, we do the same thing when we sleep. We live off our fat stores. Or we should do, but because of our confused and often incorrect information about how, what and when to eat, we actually stop our bodies from using up those fat stores at night, so we deny ourselves the benefits that hibernating animals get.

In fact, we humans do tend to sleep rather more in the winter than the summer. There are various theories about why this is: it may be just that we revel in the long hours of daylight and want to be up and out; it may be that we tend to feel better and more lively during the summer. It may also be that we eat a better diet in the summer.

If you were in the unlikely situation of having to tiptoe past a hibernating bear and your mobile phone gave a loud ring you would be unnecessarily frightened.

Why? Because hibernation, unlike sleep, is not easily reversible. Our sleep is very easily interrupted, but hibernation isn't. The bear, unlike you, would remain blissfully undisturbed.

The biology of sleep and hibernation look similar, are profoundly similar in their energy budgets, but also have important differences.

A sleeping bear, like us, will use fat stores for maintaining all the basic functions like heart beat, breathing and so on, and for repair, maintenance and rebuilding of new tissues.

Like us, this sleeping bear has to keep his brain function going during the night fast and like us he needs glucose to do that, so he will make sure his liver is fuelled up before he settles down for the night. The bear's sweet tooth and instinctive love of honey confirm that his brain is well aware of that need.

In theory, during hibernation a fuelled liver would be exhausted after a few hours, blood glucose would fall, the adrenal glands which pump our stress hormones would be activated and essential tissues, bone and muscle would be degraded to maintain brain function.

That's not what happens though, because the clever bear, along with other hibernating animals prevents it by converting fat stores into a special kind of fuel which the brain can use but which isn't glucose. His brain works away happily during the long winter months.

And if the brain is performing all its vital functions, overseeing all the other organs and tissues, there is no need for production of adrenal stress hormones.

Now we can clearly see the difference between hibernation and sleep: Hibernation is stress-free biology.

Sleeping without a fuelled liver is profoundly stressful for us humans. Blood glucose falls, our adrenal glands start pumping out dangerous hormones like cortisone, our muscles and bones are being degraded, our ability to fight off infection is reduced, our gut is under attack, memory cells get culled, reproductive biology is assaulted and recovery hormone production is shut down.

Nature's intention to use sleep for recovery goes into reverse and our fat stores are left undisturbed.

Every brown and black bear and every other hibernating animal know the difference between hibernation and sleep, no stress and high stress. Somehow we humans haven't really grasped the concept yet.

Hibernating animals feed themselves up during the season of plenty, stacking up lots of extra weight for the period in which they will put themselves into just-ticking-over mode. It's a superb mechanism for dealing with long periods when food is hard to get and breeding isn't necessary. As an energy-efficiency exercise, hibernation is the ultimate exemplar.

As humans, there's quite a lot we can learn from animals like some bears, rodents, insects, badgers, hedgehogs and others who either go into full hibernation or into a dorm-ant state over winter. Their body temperature falls, breath-ing slows, they give up on certain ordinary functions for a few months, and their heart beat slows down. They need the minimal level of nutrients to tick over because the demands on their bodies are minimised. They live off stored fat and get up in the spring starving but healthy.

Hormones and resistance

Complicated things, hormones. They behave differently in the two genders; they dictate everything from growth to reproduction, happiness to depression, stress to content-ment. They are not universally delightful items though. There are adrenal hormones. These are the ones that cause stress, make us panic, pump out stimulating effects and then leave our brutalised bodies to pick up the pieces. They make us sweat at night, leave us feeling tired when we get up, cause sudden changes in blood sugar levels, affect our mood and cause total fatigue. The Hibernation Diet shows you how to avoid producing them by making sure your body is not deprived of vital fuel during the night.

The exercise component in the Hibernation Diet isn't what you'll be familiar with. It isn't about pounding it out in the gym or doing exhausting exercise classes. Instead, we suggest – but we don't compel – that you do some resistance exercises.

This form of exercise activates production of recovery hormones during Slow Wave Sleep and recovery is exclusively fat-burning biology.

But what exactly is resistance exercise? It just means using your muscles to counter some kind of resistance. It might be pushing a chair nearer the television, lifting a milk bottle out of the fridge, or raising and lowering a one kilogram weight in each hand.

What the Hibernation Diet recommends is that you conscientiously include two or three bursts of resistance exercise each week. You don't need to join a gym to do it. You can buy light hand weights or use, say, packs of sugar, rice or dried beans. Use the resistance of your own body in exercises with these with a fit ball for example. Yoga, Pilates, cycling and floor exercises – there are many videos and DVDs available – are all resistance exercises. We have included a short resistance exercise routine for you a little further on – see Join the Heroic Resistance Movement on p.43.

For those of you who enjoy the gym, then we'll show you how to make it work better for you. For those of you who hate it, or are perhaps feeling too fragile for that kind of exercise, we'll give you easy-to-follow alternatives.

But although your weight loss may be slower without exercise, it will still happen and you will still feel a hundred times healthier and fitter than you do at the moment.

'TIRED ALL THE TIME'

Why do we complain about being tired all the time? It's a distress signal, an SOS, a warning that, without action, there could be a crisis up ahead.

Our bodies can store only small amounts of usable energy, and our brains can't store any.

So what's the answer? The Hibernation Diet, a new lifestyle, will allow your body to maximise its own potential and you will feel the benefits.

We'll show you how to exploit your own natural resources and make your body work for your physical and mental well-being without having to torture yourself in the gym or follow difficult and dangerous faddish diet regimes.

When you see the Hibernation Diet working, you'll discover that not only do you feel so much better, fitter, more energetic, but you will also realise your body had resources that you never knew about before. You'll be able to manage your life, with all its demands, much better than you ever thought possible, and you'll look and feel great too.

We'll teach you what the sources of your fatigue are and how to get rid of them. We'll show you the damage that you're doing to your own body's biology and how to change that. We'll teach you how easy it is to say goodbye to feeling tired and drained and hello to health and vitality.

So the principles of this new lifestyle are:

- **Going to bed with enough fuel in your liver to feed your brain**
- **Using honey as the fuelling mechanism at night**
- **Making sure you get enough quality sleep**
- **Eating holistically and avoiding highly refined or processed foods**
- **Undertaking some short, sharp bursts of**

'push/pull' resistance work for maximum results
- Exploiting your own body's capacity to burn up your fat reserves

HIBERNATION HONEY AT NIGHT

Take a generous tablespoonful of honey at night, either in a warm drink, a smoothie or straight from the jar. See the recipes on p. 38 for honey drinks.

What's so special about honey?

Honey has the same amounts of glucose and fructose.

So?

Your liver takes in the fructose.

The fructose regulates glucose into the liver.

That keeps your blood sugar level balanced all night.

No sudden highs or sudden lows.

Your liver has stores to keep your brain fuelled.

You don't need to release dangerous stress hormones. Your recovery hormones get on with their job ...

... and they use up your fat stores to do it.

NIGHT NONSENSE

There is a myth that you should never eat at night. It's really bad for you. Your food just lies in your stomach and turns to fat because you're not doing anything. And everyone knows your metabolic rate falls overnight, so you can't burn any calories. Anyway, you can't sleep properly on a full stomach.

Now, we're not going to give you *carte blanche* to stuff yourself with takeaways every night. We're talking here about nutrition; about giving your body the right fuel to work with.

SARAH, THE NIGHT RAIDER

Sarah was fit and healthy, working and running after her two children. She was heavier than she wanted to be, in spite of being a member of a gym and exercising around six hours a week on a cardiovascular workout. She'd come home from the gym, feed the kids and herself, do all the essential tasks that crowded her day, and fall into bed.

But Sarah kept on waking up consumed with hunger, raiding the fridge on a regular basis at about one or two in the morning. She'd gobble up the children's leftovers, tuck into carb and sugar-rich foods, and head back to bed.

In the morning, she had a headache and felt rotten.

The Hibernation Diet answers

We encouraged Sarah away from her running and aerobics classes on to a resistance-based regime using her own body weight to exercise. She would do two or three 15-minute sessions a week using gym equipment such as the leg press and arm curls. She'd also use a fit ball and do floor exercises. We suggested a bedtime snack, but Sarah said, 'Oh no, eat before bed? That makes you fatter!'

We explained how fuelling up her liver before bed with a natural fructose based snack would optimise her fat burning potential. She'd have a stable blood glucose level overnight – important for all of us because peaks and troughs have debilitating side-effects even for non-diabetics – and would wake up slimmer, more energetic, and in a better state of repair. 'Okay, I'll buy that!' And she did. Off she went with a couple of pots of honey in hand. Sarah soon learned the benefits of fuelling the liver with honey before bed. Not only did she lose weight, she awoke in the mornings bursting with fresh energy.

MORNING SICKNESS

While we're demolishing myths, let's deal with the one about skipping breakfast. We've all heard: 'I never eat breakfast'. 'I can't eat in the morning.' 'The thought of food makes me feel sick until about lunchtime.'

But lots of us know that if we force down a slice of toast in the morning, we'll definitely feel better. Why is that?

It's the liver again. A slice of toast with fruit juice replenishes our liver and stabilises blood glucose. We stop producing the nauseating stress hormones and start to feel more normal.

Morning sickness is caused by low blood glucose and whether you're pregnant or not, male or female, low blood glucose is dangerous. If you're driving, operating machinery, or just asleep in bed, low blood glucose throws your body into serious panic, pumping out hormones for all it's worth, and leaving behind damaging after-effects.

All you need to do to avoid it is to fuel up your liver before you sleep. It's simple, easy and cheap. And by the way, it's even more vital if you've been drinking alcohol, which pushes your blood glucose level down during the night, the main reason for a hangover.

Now let's take a look at another simple foundation stone that plays a vital part in the Hibernation Diet.

We've already talked quite a lot about sleep: Slow Wave Sleep, those hormones produced during sleep, bad sleep, night-time hunger and low levels of glucose in the blood during sleep.

But what about the quality of our sleep?

From the days of our caveman ancestors right up until the early twentieth century, night time was dark! Even with candles and the light from a fire, we were not surrounded by bright light. Now, we are. Street lighting, car lights, even the small electronic lights from the television, computer or other LEDs, permeate day and night.

In some countries, lights are used as torture, forcing prisoners into surrender. It is a rare reality to experience truly total darkness.

Light pollution doesn't just stop us from enjoying the night sky. It damages nature too.

A trainer told us about his father who worked in the oil industry in the Far East.

When a flare pipe was put up close to a rice crop, the crop failed to thrive, even though the light and heat were too high up to alter the ground temperature.

The farmers noticed that where the crops were shielded from the light, they did thrive. The light that fractured the dark period in the light/dark cycle of the rice was causing the damage. The crop was confused.

We have a small gland in the brain, called the pineal, known as the 'third eye'. It reacts to light changes, releasing the hormone, melatonin, when darkness falls. This sleep hormone needs total darkness to bring all the benefits of sleep recovery and to optimise our fat-burning opportunities.

So get rid of any artificial light source from your bedroom.

SLOW WAVE SLEEP

So now we've got fuelling up our liver before sleep and keeping the bedroom dark. Is there anything else we can do to make sure we optimise all the fat-burning and repair work that Slow Wave Sleep can bring?

JENNY'S MIDDAY SIESTA

Jenny, a thirty-something accountant, was a recreational exerciser, a keep fit fanatic who exercised most evenings for around 90 minutes and also ran for 30–40 minutes at lunchtime packing in a quick sandwich before going back to her desk.

She was permanently exhausted. We had previously suggested fuelling correctly pre-exercise in the evening and refuelling her liver with honey before bed. She had taken our advice and felt so good and energetic that she added the lunchtime run to her regime. She had returned complaining again of physical and emotional exhaustion.

The Hibernation Diet Answer

We suggested she take a lunchtime nap for half an hour, eating half her lunch from our Eating Outlines (p. 00) before the nap and the other half afterwards. We explained how that would release recovery hormones, calming down her stress level, and setting her up for the busy afternoon ahead.

Refuelling her liver would cut back on the emotional rollercoaster effect, giving her a sense of calm and well-being for the rest of the day.

'Just like the Spanish!' she said. 'The siesta is a great concept!' She never looked back.

Sleep burns fat if you provide the body with the repairing incentive to do it. Your body loves to sacrifice fat to perform recovery work. All we have to do is make sure that it has the materials and a good working environment that includes stable blood glucose and no stress hormones pumping out, and it will return the compliment with the very gift you seek. And some!

Good quality sleep also has a big impact upon the ageing process, so if you would like to try to hold it back, read on to find out more about Slow Wave Sleep and why it matters so much.

Age comes to all of us, no matter how hard we try to fight it off. The biggest killer in today's westernised society is still heart disease and the lifestyle problems that lead to it: high cholesterol levels, hardened arteries, obesity, sedentary lifestyle, too much alcohol and of course smoking, still the biggest killer we have to tackle.

Because we're getting fatter, because we're getting less active, we're hastening our own death, and even though, on average, we are living longer because of medical advances in areas like the control of bacterial infection, drug treatments and advances in sophisticated forms of surgery, a lot of what kills us lies within our own control to change.

It's in the simple areas like how we eat, sleep and live – but we ignore the obvious in favour of the obscure.

Hang on, are you trying to tell me that it's within my own power to hold back the ageing process?

We have a powerful anti-ageing option already built into our recovery biology that we talked about earlier. It's Slow Wave Sleep. You may have heard of it. That's where our capacity to rebuild and replenish all the older tissue lies; our chance, if you like, to defy age.

Come on, aren't we all just going to get old and die? I mean, we're all disintegrating, aren't we? Our brain cells die off at some incredible rate every day after we're about 25, so any notion of somehow defying that has to be nonsense. That'd be the Holy Grail.

Do you know about the Second Law of Thermodynamics? That's the idea that we're all slowly disintegrating, that entropy or decay is as integral to humans as it is to everything else in the universe, from polystyrene cups to biodegradable toilet paper. But we humans keep on renewing ourselves. We're an offence to that Second Law because we're organised, dynamic, replenishing, rebuilding all the time. We're a total contradiction.

And Slow Wave Sleep is when we do all that stuff? When we rebuild ourselves in that recovery biology period you're talking about? So we're really reversing nature in a way?

Reversing, yes, we can say that. We are reversing the natural process of decay and disintegration. We are holding back time.

So if I've got this straight, what you're saying is that if we work towards optimising that recovery process in Slow Wave Sleep, then we are in a kind of time dilation, aren't we?

We're not promising the key to eternal life. We haven't found the Holy Grail just yet, but what we are saying is that if we move in tune with our own cyclical rhythms, our own biological music if you like, then we can certainly make the natural melodies work for us.

What else can we do to help move things along?

HEROIC RESISTANCE EXERCISE

We've already mentioned resistance exercise. Let's now look at it more closely. The trend for fitness and health has emphasised aerobic exercise – the kind that makes your heart work harder, gets you hot and panting – and, we're told, burns up calories.

This kind of exercise is good for our general fitness – because it helps to lower blood pressure and improve stamina but the idea that it will burn off a lot of calories is a bit misleading.

In fact, when you're fighting for your breath on a run and your body needs energy to keep going, a lot of it comes from your muscles. Breaking down muscle to get calories isn't what you need to lose weight. You need to burn your fat stores.

It is not vital that you include resistance exercise. The Hibernation Diet will work without it, but adding in resistance workouts will certainly speed up your weight loss and improve your flexibility and general health. Resistance kicks the process into overdrive, giving your body an extra incentive to work harder at night on that repair and recovery. That means burning more night calories, so it speeds up weight loss.

If you do include it, and it's your decision, then check first with your doctor, especially if you suffer from any pre-existing medical condition such as back problems, heart problems, arthritis or rheumatism.

If you intend to go to the gym, then find yourself a good, qualified personal trainer to draw up a suitable programme that meets your uniquely individual needs. If you plan to exercise alone, then refer to Join the Heroic Resistance Movement p. 43.

Resistance exercise is much safer than suddenly taking up running on a treadmill for an hour a day, for example, and can be easily matched to your own age, size and strength. But the decision is yours, and even without intensifying the benefits in this way, the Hibernation Diet will still change your life.

Healthy Eating

Most of the current diet fashions centre only on what we eat. Atkins told us to eat lots of fat and protein but no carbohydrates. The GI Diet is based around foods with a low glycaemic index which slowly raise our blood glucose levels and take longer to digest, using up some calories in the process. There have been fad diets like the combination diet, cabbage diet, grapefruit diet, hard boiled egg diet, all of which focus on particular foods or food groups.

But eating healthily isn't about excluding whole food groups. It's about eating a well balanced mixture of wholesome foods that provide the nutrients we all need without overloading our systems with unnecessary additives.

Again, it's where the Hibernation Diet focuses on common sense and our own biology. We don't want to starve you, we don't want to wear you out with pounding a treadmill, we don't want you to suffer from indigestion and bad breath, and we don't want you to have to deny yourself the foods you enjoy.

You don't need to. Far from it. Our philosophy is based on natural, healthy eating, so ditch the pre-packed dinners, nutrition-less white bread, endless colourings and flavourings, and buy foods that your body will like.

BODY-FRIENDLY FOODS

Increasingly, supermarkets are storing organic produce in response to demand, but do seek out local suppliers in the smaller shops and local markets. There are also some good online organic suppliers of meat, fish, vegetables and other products. Far better to shop three times a week, buying smaller quantities that are ultra-fresh, than buy everything at once.

THE FOOD QUIZ

What do you know about the food you eat? Try this quiz to test out your knowledge.

1. Which of these foods is highest in carbohydrates?
   a. A slice of fruit cake
   b. A flapjack
   c. A slice of Battenburg cake

2. Which of these kinds of bread contains most fibre?
   a. A slice of granary bread
   b. Half a plain Naan
   c. A slice of sourdough bread

3. Which of these foods has the lowest glycaemic index (GI)?
   a. Potato
   b. Chocolate
   c. Porridge oats

4. Gram for gram, which of these foods is richest in protein?
   a. Lamb's liver

b. Dry roasted peanuts
c. Cheddar cheese

5. To retain the vitamins in vegetables, are you better to:
   a. Steam them
   b. Microwave them
   c. Boil them?

6. Which of these nutrients is vital for maintaining a strong immune system?
   a. Iron
   b. Vitamin C
   c. Zinc

7. Which of these three most benefit from protein in our diet?
   a. Our energy resources
   b. Our hair
   c. Our hormone production

8. Which of these foods makes you feel the fullest?
   a. Carrots
   b. Steak
   c. Chips

Answers:

(1) Yes, they're all pretty heavy but you might be surprised to know that the Battenburg, with 52.7g in every 100g is even worse than the fruit cake at 43.4g. At least the fruit cake has a few good ingredients, but a supermarket-bought Battenburg is packed with highly refined flour, sugar, cheap saturated fat and colourings. The flapjack comes in at 45.3g but does have a low GI and is full of natural ingredients.

(2) Bread is a daily source of fibre for most of us and, generally, the best sources are wholegrain and wholemeal breads. A slice of granary comes in at 3.8g per 100g. The Naan sounds better than most white bread at 2.0g but that's misleading because it is also

heavy in added fat. Sourdough bread has virtually no fibre (0.9g). Oh, and just being brown doesn't equal high fibre, so check the nutrition content label.

(3) This is a bit of a trick question. The GI index is usually a safe way to compare how quickly or slowly foods break down and raise your blood sugar level – the slower the better. But some foods with low GI are not the ones to have too much of in your diet. Chocolate has the lowest GI, but don't be tempted to cut out potatoes or oatmeal in its favour.

(4) Protein is vital to our body for energy and essential cell building. A small portion of fried lamb's liver, just 100g, contains 30.1g of protein. Dry roasted peanuts, though they do contain a massive 51.2g per 100g, don't include some of the other rich nutrients like iron that liver does and are heavy in calorie content. Cheese has 25.6g of protein per 100g.

(5) Microwave them to retain the maximum nutritional value. Best of all, buy a microwave steamer. You can steam them on the hob of course, but please avoid boiling them and removing most of the valuable ingredients.

(6) All of them in different ways.

(7) Hormone production, for which the protein provides nitrogen to make hormones.

(8) Carrots. The reason is that carrot contains the perfect balance of glucose and fructose for your liver and brain. Once your liver is well fuelled, the brain relaxes and reduces your urge to eat more.

THE HIBERNATION DIET FOOD CIRCLE

You may well be familiar with the main food groups, but here's a good old-fashioned, non-faddish reminder of what they are and what they do:

Proteins are life's building materials. They're essential for skin, cells, enzymes, hormones. All the things that make life possible. Main sources are milk (also useful for calcium), eggs, cheese, soya, fish, meat and poultry.

Carbohydrates have been given a bad reputation, quite wrongly. They're essential for energy and to keep blood glucose levels stable, especially during physical activity. The brain needs carbs to function. The problems come when we fill up with highly refined white sugar and bread. We need to focus on carbs that contain fructose as well as glucose because the fructose releases the carbs for the brain to take them up. The best and oldest source for that one-to-one balance is honey. The ancient Egyptians knew that but we've forgotten it. The most important carbohydrates are fruits and vegetables because they contain a one-to-one balance of glucose and fructose, the perfect ratio for fuelling the liver, supplying the brain and achieving stable blood glucose levels.

Fats fall into two groups: saturated and unsaturated. Animal fats are saturated: the body doesn't really need them, and they get stored in layers of fatty tissue, increase cholesterol that clogs up our arteries and increases the risk of heart disease. Unsaturated fats are good guys that come from oily fish and some plant oils. They contain vital omega 3 and omega 6 oils. That's why olive oil is good but lard is bad!

Vitamins and minerals Vitamins are essential to every cell within our bodies. We get them from dietary sources of all sorts. We can't produce them ourselves, so we need to make sure that we choose foods that provide rich natural sources of these crucial nutrients. Minerals are indeed the very elements we learned about in chemistry. They form in the planet first in plant sources; animals eat plants, and we either eat the animals or the animals slowly disintegrate and merge into the earth's crust, complete with minerals. As with vitamins, we can't make our own, so rely on our diet to get them. Highly processed supermarket meals, takeaways and other kinds of fast food lose most of these nutrients in the preparation, so it makes sense to supplement where necessary.

GOLDEN RULES

Lean meat eaten three or four times a week is good. If you're vegetarian, you'll need to include lots of soya and other protein alternatives.

Fish is fab because it contains virtually no fat (except the good kinds in oily fish), is a cinch to cook, and offers loads of variety. It's an incredibly rich source of protein and a whole stack of essential vitamins and minerals. Don't overcook it and eat a mixture of oily and non-oily types. Oily fish are anchovy, herring, mackerel, pilchards, sardines, tuna, whitebait, trout, salmon. The rest are mainly what you will think of as white fish: brill, flounder, halibut, plaice, sole, bass, bream, cod, coley, haddock, hake, monkfish, whiting.

Eggs are a convenient source of protein, but don't overdo your intake of them because they may raise cholesterol. Two or three a week is enough.

Carbohydrates should be eaten every day, making sure you balance the sources between bread and pasta with fructose-filled fruits, vegetables and honey so that you always have fuel for your brain.

GO SHOPPING

You're starting up a whole new lifestyle. Clean out your store cupboards, get rid of goods you now know have no place in your Hibernation Diet future. Head out to the local shops for some really fresh, good, ideally organic products to get you on your way. We're not excluding you from the supermarkets, but check labels, seek out the freshest and don't buy anything that's highly processed, full of colours and preservatives, and won't contribute to your wellbeing. Avoid buying bigger quantities than you need. Fresh food, even though it may still be usable after several days, loses a lot of its natural nutrition with storage.

So look for seasonal veg and fruit that's fresh and firm. If it's out of season, it will probably have been grown in heated greenhouses where, again, it loses a lot of its nutritional value. If you have a local Farmers' Market or indeed any kind of market, you'll get fresher and cheaper produce than at the supermarket. Buy lots of fresh fruit - any kind that you like – and do include potatoes.

Buy fish that looks really wet and fresh. It's a food that is so much better from your local fishmonger than your local supermarket. No matter how hard they try, supermarket fish just never looks as fresh and natural. Besides, local fishmongers will have more variety and will stock locally caught fresh fish. They'll also fillet it for you if you ask.

Local butchers seem to be almost as much a dying breed as their traditional stock these days, with pre-packed meat in polystyrene containers topped with clingfilm taking over from well-hung sides and meat that didn't have red colourings added to it. But if you can find one, do use it and seek out meat that is freshly cut and looks it.

Some butchers will even trim off fat for you if you ask. Some also store good fresh poultry as well, so check that out. If you just can't access meat other than from a supermarket, look online for organic producers who will deliver to your door.

When it comes to carbs, beware the fresh scent of baking in the supermarket. These delightful looking baguettes and bagels are mostly produced from pre-mixes supplied to the outlet and then mixed with water. They contain highly refined white flour, saturated fats, dried yeast and preservatives, colourings and flavourings. Your body takes a look, doesn't see much that's of any use, and deposits the leftovers as fatty tissue just in case there's a famine ahead and you'll need the stores.

For dairy products, there are now good organic cheese makers all over the country, so enjoy their produce (but not too much because they are high in calories). Organic milk is now readily available in supermarkets and contains extra nutrients, but you don't need to buy full-fat milk to benefit from these unless you are buying for growing children. Natural and fruit yoghurts are good and better if organic, but avoid the sticky sugar-filled varieties.

Store cupboard goods will last longer than fresh foods of course. Make sure you get that crucial honey and try to avoid using white sugar. Products like Marmite are useful as a rich source of the essential B vitamins. Nuts, dried fruit, mixed seeds, pulses, all offer good snack foods. Buy omega-rich oils like olive and sesame and keep them in a cool, dark place to preserve their goodness. Pasta and rice are convenient and readily available. Look for wholegrain varieties and brown or wild rice for preference. Wholegrain crispbreads are useful.

A WORD ABOUT COOKING

Preparing and cooking of your food makes a huge difference to how much good it does you. If you over-boil vegetables, bake fish too long or deep-fry poultry, then you're effectively destroying its valuable nutritional benefits.

So once you've purchased lean cuts of meat, good quality poultry and fresh vegetables, don't wipe out all your good work in the kitchen.

By all means add fresh herbs, pepper and seasoning, but go easy on salt. Trim off any fat from meat and skin poultry (it's all right to do this after you've cooked it).

Use a meat thermometer to check roasting meat and to avoid overcooking it. Fish needs very little cooking time.

THE HIBERNATION HONEY-EATING PLAN

Are you ready for this? We thought we'd give you a few statistics on that greedy brain before we set out the Honey Eating Plan.

- As you read this, your liver is emptying at the rate of 10g of glucose an hour
- About 60 per cent of that is being gobbled up by your brain so that you can see, process and mentally download the information on the page
- Your greedy brain is 2 per cent of your body, consuming 60 per cent of your available fuel from your liver
- If the rest of your body used glucose at that rate, you'd need to eat 14 loaves of bread a day just to stay alive, never mind run for the bus

So now you've a context for the enormous amount of fuel your genius furnace needs to keep going. Now let's look at how our plan works to make sure your brain is getting its goodies in the right ways and at the right times of the day.

Do pay particular attention to what we will describe as the Blue Hours. These are the times of the day when your body can slip into meltdown and you may be quite unaware of it happening beyond perhaps feeling tired and irritable. These are key points in your day.

Do drinks lots of water. It keeps your system running, helps your digestion to process and staves off any hunger pangs. Keep a bottle of water by you at all times and get into the habit of drinking regularly. You should aim to take in around two litres a day, not counting tea and coffee.

Get the Hibernation Habit: Eating Outlines

PRIME TIME 7.30–8.30 A.M.

Prime the liver, which means that fructose enters the liver and prepares it for glucose intake. Your liver is empty now and your brain is hungry because you've used up last night's honey. It's crucial that you get your liver into gear now. If you head off without a decent breakfast, you are cheating yourself.

You will not lose weight more quickly by starving yourself in the morning. You will be less alert, less aware of traffic, more likely to step off the pavement in front of a car, and if you're driving, more likely to cause an accident because your low blood glucose will make you a danger.

You may not feel particularly distracted or unaware, but you will be. A low blood glucose can be insidious. It can cause a headache but can itself cloud your awareness that you need fuelling. It will damage your mood for the whole day, make you feel irritable with colleagues and tired all the time.

You may feel uncomfortably sweaty, have a sense that your heart is 'fluttering', and your capacity for calm, rational analysis of work issues will be out of the window.

Choose from these breakfast options:

Apple juice
Muesli with semi-skimmed milk
Boiled egg
Low-fat yoghurt with raspberries

or   Tomato juice
Porridge with semi-skimmed milk
1 poached egg
Fresh orange juice
2 rashers of grilled bacon on one slice wholemeal toast

or   Fruit salad of sliced apple and orange
Bran flakes with semi-skimmed milk
1 poached egg

or   Fresh orange juice
1 slice wholegrain bread spread with olive tapenade
A portion of low-fat cheese
2 plums

or   1 banana
1 slice wholegrain bread with low-fat spread and topped with lean ham
Low-fat yoghurt with 2 teaspoonfuls of honey

or   Honey (2 teaspoons) in herbal tea
Muesli with low fat milk
1 boiled egg and 1 slice wholemeal toast and low-fat spread
Fruit salad of sliced pear and orange

or   Tomato juice
Grilled bacon and egg with beans
1 slice toasted wholegrain bread and honey
Strawberries with low-fat yoghurt

INBETWEEN TIME 10.30–11.30 A.M.

Choose from:

> A small handful of nuts/seeds/dried fruit
> A piece of (any) fruit
> A few wholegrain bread stick snacks
> A multigrain bar containig honey

LUNCH TIME 12.30–1.30 P.M.

If you're in the habit of buying a sandwich at work, we'd like to suggest you save money and know better what you're eating by making it yourself! If you live close to work, or work at home, you may be able to grab a short nap. If you can, it'll transform your afternoon and you'll find yourself far more productive. Even lying back in a chair and dozing for 10 or 15 minutes will make a real difference because you give your hormones a little time to do some repair and maintenance at the mid-point of your day.

Choose from:

> Orange juice
> 2 slices wholegrain bread with olive oil spread or olive oil for dipping, with a tuna filling and cold grilled mushrooms and cucumber
> Sliced apple with low-fat cheese

or Fruit salad of sliced apple and orange segments
> Basmati rice with lean ham, and salad of tomatoes, beans and cabbage leaves
> 1 multigrain bar (no added sugar)

or Tomato juice
Couscous with sardines, asparagus, onions and
mushrooms
Low-fat cheese
2 plums

or Fruit juice
Wholemeal bread with olive oil
Pasta with herring, onions, cucumber and lettuce
Strawberries with low-fat yoghurt

or Raspberries in low-fat yoghurt
Mixed bean salad with olive bruschetta
Low-fat cheese with 1 oatcake
1 banana

or Orange juice
2 wholegrain slices bread with lean pork and a
salad of cucumber, lettuce, cherry tomatoes
A small portion of low-fat cheese and a few dates

or 1 pineapple slice
Portion of penne pasta with lean chicken, mung
beans and mushrooms
2 oatcakes with low-fat cheese

BLUE TIME ONE… At the end of your working day

Back in the dim and distant more leisurely and
Bohemian past, artists and writers gathered on the Left
Bank of the Seine in Paris to discuss the day at around 5
p.m. or so. They'd have a coffee or a glass of wine and
perhaps a snack of oysters or snails (well, sometimes).
We're so rushed these days, we don't try to fit this in,
but we'd all benefit from what Winnie-the-Pooh would
have called 'a little something' at this time of the day.

Indeed, Pooh's honey choice would be ideal just to top up your liver before you get home and begin cooking a proper meal.

Choose from:

> A small packet of dry roasted peanuts
> A banana
> Two crispbreads with low-fat cheese or honey

BLUE TIME TWO ... When you arrive home

Depending how long it takes you to get home, you may be prone to fall into that trap of pouring a drink and flopping down on the sofa with a packet of crisps before doing anything. If you are, you're asking for trouble. Any alcohol you consume will be pushing your blood glucose down while the fast-food snack is trying to push it up. Your system is in total confusion. You'll doze for a while, wake up starving, and start the whole thing again. If this sounds familiar, do repeat the main Blue Hour snack when you get home. You'll be amazed how much less tired you'll feel, how you will enjoy your kids, partner and general conversation instead of feeling irritable and exhausted.

Choose from:

> Grated carrot with raisins

or Beetroot with cucumber or tomato

or Artichoke in unsaturated oil

or Two oatcakes with sun-dried tomatoes

or Sliced tomatoes with low-fat cheese and black pepper

or One wholegrain slice of toasted bread with olive oil
and peppers

or Sliced apple with cucumber and low-fat cheese

DINNER TIME 6.30–8 P.M.

For most of us, this is the main meal of the day, and it will
often have to consider the demands of other people.
Children can be choosy and partners not much less so. Our
suggestions are flexible enough to fit around the preferences you have to deal with, especially if you're the one
doing the cooking.

Your evening meal should be rich in vital nutrients and
contain lots of fresh fruit/vegetables, but it should not
leave you feeling heavy and bloated. Be careful about
portion size and do try to take a walk or do a little resistance work a couple of hours later.

Choose from

Tomato juice
Home-made vegetable soup (potato, leek, tomato
or mushroom and a small portion of low-fat cheese
Grilled herring, boiled new potatoes in skins,
carrots, cabbage, peppers, onions
Low-fat yoghurt with strawberries

or Orange juice
Mixed leaf salad with mung beans, pinto beans,
cucumber, lettuce, peppers, green olives
Sirloin steak grilled, basmati rice, mushrooms,
onions, carrots
Sliced melon with ginger

or 1 pineapple slice

Vegetable soup with tomato, onions, broccoli, carrots
Roast organic chicken with cabbage, cauliflower, spinach and roasted potatoes
Salad of fresh fruit with honey

or   Tomato juice
Grilled fresh tuna (or tinned in sunflower oil) with noodles, peppers, butter beans
Low-fat cheese with oatcakes
Raspberries in low-fat yoghurt

or   Tomato and basil salad with 1 teaspoon of olive oil and vinegar
Ham, avocado, mushrooms and onions
2 teaspoonfuls honey in low-fat yoghurt

or   Mango juice
Small salad of low-fat cheese, (cubed) apple, dates and cherry tomatoes
Roast lamb, couscous, peppers, broccoli and carrots
Fruit sorbet

or   Orange, cucumber and avocado salad
Roast organic turkey, boiled potatoes in skin, carrots, onions, butter beans
Apricots and low-fat yoghurt

BED TIME

No choices. It's HONEY. One or two tablespoons in the hour before you go to bed

But certainly vary the way you take your tablespoon of honey (two, if you're larger than average) by adding hot water, lemon, cloves or putting it into a cup of peppermint

tea or camomile tea for example. Alternatively, choose
from one of the smoothie recipes provided below. Spread
it on a slice of toast or a couple of crispbreads for a change,
or put it into a pot of low-fat plain yoghurt. However you
choose to take it, the honey is vital to store up your liver an
hour or so before you sleep.

You'll sleep restfully while your body will be busily
burning up your excess fat, and carrying out its maintenance and repair programme uninterrupted by stress
hormones. You won't just be dreaming about being
slimmer and healthier, that's exactly what will be happening. You are recovering, devouring up those extra fat stores
while the fructose is busily cleaning out toxins.

HIBERNATION HONEY DRINKS

Here's a variety of honey-based drinks that you can enjoy
at any time to give yourself a nutritional lift and to fuel up
your liver and brain. You can vary them using your own
tastes and preferences, and they're an ideal way to take
your night-time honey.

Honey and banana smoothie

$1/2$ cup of low-fat milk
1 medium or 2 small bananas, cut roughly
$1/2$ cup of plain low-fat yoghurt
$1/4$ cup of honey
Dash of vanilla essence.
A pinch each of around cinnamon and nutmeg
Add ice and blend until smooth

Strawberry and honey smoothie

>1 cup of low fat vanilla ice cream
>1 cup of strawberries
>$^1/_4$ cup of low-fat milk
>$^1/_4$ cup of honey
>Add ice and blend until smooth

Honey and fruit thirst quencher

>2 teaspoons of honey
>Pinch of salt
>2 cups of any natural fruit juice or blend of juices
>$^1/_2$ cup of tepid water
>Add ice and blend until smooth

Honey latte

>1 cup of coffee (warm or cold)
>$^1/_2$ cup of low fat milk (warm or cold)
>2 teaspoons of honey
>Blend or stir through.
>Add ice to the cold version and blend

Winter honey punch

>1 cup of dry cider
>$^1/_2$ cup of cranberry juice
>2 teaspoons of honey
>Pinch of cinnamon
>Warm all the ingredients together in a saucepan,
>but do not boil

Honey breakfast refresher

> 1 cup of low-fat yoghurt
> 2 teaspoons of honey
> $1/2$ cup of fresh orange juice
> One banana
> Blend all ingredients together until smooth and add ice

Herbal teas

These are another great way of satisfying thirst without adding unwelcome sugars and stimulants. There are lots of proprietary brands available, but you can easily create your own.

Energising herbal teas such as Ginseng, Rhodiola, Rooibos, Tangerine, and Ginger may be taken with honey in the morning or for energy during the day.

Detoxifying teas may be taken with honey on the morning after and include Milk Thistle, Liquorice, Ginger, Sage, Peppermint, Spearmint, Burdock and Dandelion. The honey adds another wonderful power punch to the detoxifying process.

Soothing teas may be taken with honey during the day and include Peach, Rosehip, Cinnamon and Hibiscus.

Calming herbal teas to be taken late in the evening to prepare for the night fast and for Slow Wave Sleep include Lime Flowers, Valerian, Fennel, Hops, Chamomile, Rosehips and Cinnamon.

Pick your herbs according to the time of day and your particular situation. Use boiling water and let it cool naturally, or chill and ice the teas you make.

Add 2 teaspoons of honey to each cup measure you make.

Simple Simon

Boiling water, two teaspoons of honey and a pinch each of ginger and cinnamon. A light, tasty and healthy start to the day. Ginger gives a great enthusiasm burst that drives up motiviation.

Punch Up

Boiling water, 2 teaspoons of honey and a splash (about 1 dessertspoon full) of fresh orange juice to taste. Great Vitamin C source to start your day.

Cranberry quencher

Boiling water, 2 teaspoons of honey and 1 tablespoon of pure, fresh cranberry juice. A great pick-up and a particularly good remedy for anyone with a touch of cystitis.

Ginger up

Boiling water, 1 dessertspoon of cranberry juice, $1/2$ cup of organic ginger ale and 2 teaspoons of honey. A great energy booster that also helps to clear your mind.

Join the Heroic Resistance Movement

If you have decided that you will include some resistance work as part of your Hibernation Diet lifestyle, then this section gives you some exercises to follow. If you aren't yet sure, then here's information to help you make that choice, and if you've decided not to join the resistance movement, just go on to the next chapter!

First, though, let's take a closer look at what's involved in this kind of exercise and why it's so useful.

WHAT RESISTANCE WORK ISN'T

- It isn't body building
- It isn't a six-pack stomach
- It isn't going to make you pant and sweat.
- It isn't going to leave you feeling sore
- It isn't going to over-strain muscles
- It isn't going to involve leotards or treadmills

WHAT RESISTANCE WORK IS

In fact, resistance work is the gentlest and easiest form of exercise, and it's what we all do in minor ways every day anyway. When you lift your briefcase or shopping bag, move a chair over, go upstairs, even lift a cup of tea, you are, in a small way, doing resistance exercise because you are using your own strength against another force.

Of course, lifting cups of tea won't do much to help burn up your fat stores at night, but you can certainly use regular and concentrated short bursts to intensify the effect. You can also better use the resistance exercises you do unconsciously – so use the stairs rather than the escalator or the lift, walk to the shops rather than getting a bus, buy yourself a fit ball, discover Pilates or yoga. The options are wide.

What gives resistance exercise real effect in the Hibernation Diet are the repetitions: how often you go up and downstairs, lift the kilo hand weights, do the easy floor exercises, and how regularly. A hundred sit-ups today then none for a week won't work. But ten sit-ups each day will.

Try a little experiment. Pick up a bunch of keys. There's a small resistance. Now, using a bag if you like, take the keys, a carton of milk, a few potatoes and a small bunch of bananas and lift that. For most of us, it won't be a problem and it is probably something you do quite often. But if you now repeat that lift ten times, then by making the load greater, you have increased the resistance, and you will make a greater demand on your muscles by lifting it ten times rather than just once. You are unlikely to feel exhausted, out of breath or fit for nothing but bed.

For a few people, resistance exercise just isn't possible. Those of us who've had major surgery such as hip or knee replacements may lack the flexibility. Serious arthritic conditions can cause problems, although gentle resistance can also help some of those who suffer from arthritis and rheumatism. If you have in the past, or have recently, suffered an injury, then that may rule out exercise at least for a time. But for most of us, gentle resistance exercise is good not only for increasing weight loss but for general flexibility.

Yoga is a good form of resistance, as is Pilates, and these are, by their very nature, gentle and tuned to your own degree of movement and flexibility. You gradually add greater resistance as you become accustomed to each level of effort, so making your muscles stronger.

But, for the Hibernation Diet, the crucial point about resistance exercise is that it so effectively accelerates your body's ability to carry out that night-time recovery and maintenance work that we've already mentioned a few times. To strengthen muscles, your body releases recovery hormones, and they're the good guys that work at using up your fat during the night. All these recovery hormones are the very same ones that burn fat while you sleep. You could perhaps call them the Hibernation Hormones!

THE BENEFITS OF RESISTING

What resistance exercise can do for you:

- Improve your posture
- Make you more supple
- Trim your shape
- Tone your muscles
- Slow down ageing
- Accelerate fat loss
- Improve your mood
- Improve your metabolism
- Cut back stress hormones
- Increase bone density
- Relieve arthritic joints
- Aid digestion
- Lower blood pressure

- Help low back pain
- Relieve depression
- Increase bone strength in older people
- Improve sleep

You might have noticed that these benefits coincide with those of the Hibernation Diet. The remarkable thing is, though, that the Hibernation Diet will still deliver these results even without resistance exercise. But this gentle form of exercising will add to the benefits and give you that great bonus of increased fat-burning at night.

But why will it happen?

Resistance exercises release the recovery hormones, those hormones that only burn fats, more active.

So doing this kind of exercise will make your body's recovery hormones more active at night. Your metabolic rate will increase during that four hours of Slow Wave Sleep. Even later in the night, when you sleep more lightly, you'll be burning more of your fat stores.

It'll enhance the effect of waking up. You'll feel lighter, trimmer, more energetic and more supple.

And there's more: these recovery hormones are global hormones. What does that mean? It means that they act on every single organ and tissue in your body. So if you've injured your ankle or hurt your knee, broken your leg even, then the fact that you can still do resistance exercise on your upper body while sitting down will stimulate the recovery in the broken leg. You're not only losing fat, you're helping the healing process too.

THE HOME RESISTANCE MOVEMENT

Here is a selection of gentle resistance exercises that you can do at home and which don't need complicated or expensive equipment. Even with these, if you have even a shadow of doubt, check with your doctor. If you can get a qualified personal trainer to run through them once with you, then you will be confident that you are on safe ground.

Dress comfortably in loose clothing. You can either wear trainers or go barefoot, whichever feels easier for you. Make sure the floor surface is non-slip and that you have a solid dining chair to sit on and use to help your balance. It's better to decide on specific times of the day, morning or evening, to carry out your two 15-minute sessions and stick as closely as possible to that. Leave at least an hour after eating. We recommend that you aim to take this mini-workout at 11 a.m. and 9 p.m. each day.

THE RESISTANCE ROUTINE: THREE TIMES WEEKLY FOR 15–30 MINUTES

These exercises cover both the lower and upper body and should be carried out in the sequence given here.

Exercise 1

Sit on the chair with your feet firmly on the floor. Lean forwards and raise yourself slowly to a standing position. Don't jerk yourself up. You can use your hands as a guide as you raise and lower your body but don't lean on them. When you are standing up fully, breathe in and then slowly return to a sitting position as you exhale. You are working lots of muscle groups in both the standing up and the sitting down actions.

Repeat 10 times, building towards more repetitions according to what is comfortable for you.

Exercise 2

Now stand facing the back of the chair for balance. Slowly raise your body up on to the balls of your feet so that you are standing on your toes. Pause, count to five, breathe in and slowly return to your starting position.

Repeat 10 times, building towards more repetitions according to what is comfortable for you.

Exercise 3

Now stand in a comfortable position (away from the chair), with your feet slightly apart. Drop your arms to your sides, then swing them slowly backwards and up as far as you can comfortably manage. Don't strain! Breathe in and slowly return your arms to the starting position as you exhale.

Repeat 10 times, building towards more repetitions according to what is comfortable for you.

Exercise 4

Sit comfortably on the chair with your ankles lifted slightly off the floor. Now slowly raise your legs and flex your ankles in each direction for a count of 20. Then point your toes downwards for another count of 20. Now drop your feet comfortably back to the floor.

Repeat 10 times, building towards more repetitions according to what is comfortable for you.

Exercise 5

For this exercise you will need a tin of beans (or similar) in each hand to begin with, gradually working up to increased weights later. You can buy hand weights in different sizes from sports shops. Stand with your feet firmly planted on the floor and a little apart. Hold a weight in each hand, with your arms at your sides. Hold your head and back straight. Slowly lower your hips until they are parallel with the floor. If you can't manage this, don't worry, just go as far as is comfortable. As you repeat the exercise, your flexibility will increase. Now hold your pelvis in that position for a count of 10 and breathe in. Return to your starting position as you exhale remembering to keep your head up and your back straight.

Repeat 10 times, building towards more repetitions according to what is comfortable for you.

Exercise 6

Take the weights in each hand again and keep your arms by your sides. Move your feet slightly apart. Now, looking straight ahead and with your right leg straight, step forward with your left leg until your knee is over your left foot. Now slowly bend your right leg until your knee is almost touching the ground. Don't worry if you can't get down that far. Just go as far as you can manage. It will soon come.

Repeat 10 times, building towards more repetitions according to what is comfortable for you.

Exercise 7

Lie down flat on your back on a firm surface. Bend your knees and make sure that your feet are flat on the floor and slightly apart. Now take your weights in each hand and bring your hands to rest them on the centre of your chest with your elbows pointing outwards. Keep them level and don't let them drop downwards. Breathe in and slowly push the weights straight upwards until your arms are fully extended. Hold while you exhale. Breathe in again and bring your arms slowly downwards while you again exhale.

Repeat 10 times, building towards more repetitions according to what is comfortable for you.

Exercise 8

Take one weight in your right hand. Rest your left knee on a firm surface at a comfortable height (a solid coffee table will work if you don't have a proper gym bench), and your right foot on the floor, keeping your knee slightly bent. Now place your left hand flat on the bench/table in front of your knee. Lean forward slowly, keeping your right foot firmly on the floor, and bring your right arm down from chest height until you have fully extended it in front of you. Pause for a count of five, breathe in and gradually raise the weight, keeping your arm extended, until it reaches your chest again. Slowly return to your starting position.

Repeat 10 times, building towards more repetitions according to what is comfortable for you. Then repeat the exercise with the weight in your left hand.

Exercise 9

With a weight in each hand, stand comfortably with your feet slightly apart and your arms by your sides. Breathe in, and using a forward motion, slowly bring the weights up to shoulder height as you breathe out, keeping your elbows tucked into each side. Keep your head and back straight. Hold for a count of five. Take another deep breath in and gradually lower the weights back to your starting position.

Repeat 10 times, building towards more repetitions according to what is comfortable for you.

Exercise 10

Place your right knee on a low bench or suitable, stable alternative, with your right hand flat on the bench in front of your knee. Take a weight in your left hand, turning it towards your body while keeping your hand level with your hip and your elbow tucked into your side. Breathe in, and gradually extend your left arm outwards in front of you as you breathe out, pushing the weight forward. Pause and count to five, breathe in as you return your arm to the starting position.

Repeat 10 times, building towards more repetitions according to what is comfortable for you.

Exercise 11

Sit on a firm chair (a dining room chair is fine) with your feet firmly on the floor and a little apart. Hold the weights in both hands, facing inwards towards your head, elbows pointing downwards. Breathe in, then stretch your arms slowly upwards as you breathe out, keeping your elbows close to your chest, until you have reached up as fully as you can while keeping your back straight. Hold for five, breathe in and slowly return to your starting position.

Repeat 10 times, building towards more repetitions according to what is comfortable for you.

Exercise 12

Stand with weights in each hand, feet slightly apart, keeping the backs of your hands facing your sides, elbows slightly bent. Breathe in and raise your arms together in front of you slowly so that, when extended, the backs of your hands are facing downwards parallel to the floor. Hold for a count of five, breathe in and slowly return to your starting position.

Repeat 10 times, building towards more repetitions according to what is comfortable for you.

ADVICE FOR GYM MEMBERS

Many of you who belong to a gym will be familiar with these kinds of resistance exercises, using different sized weights according to your personal strength and stamina.

To maximise the benefits of the Hibernation Diet, we would ask that you get your personal trainer to draw up for you an exercise plan that is strongly biased in this direction.

You will probably have a plan already, one which is more aerobic-based, and for general fitness, a little running on the treadmill, use of a stepper machine and rower, for example, are all useful. Some involve resistance too.

But please don't be conned into thinking that those are the exercises that will bring you fat loss.

Look instead to using resistance for putting your body into the right state to maximise those night-time recovery hormones.

That's the real route to weight loss.

BENEFITS FOR EVERYONE

Resistance exercise brings outstanding benefits:

- You gain strength through repetition and by gradually increasing resistance (using heavier weights)
- Your posture is improved
- You tone your muscles so that you won't tire out and you get rid of the flab
- You'll become more supple and have a trimmer shape
- You slow down the ageing process
- You get the night-time benefit of accelerating fat loss
- You'll feel much better mentally and if you have a tendency to be depressed, that will be relieved
- You'll be avoiding sudden blood glucose level changes that can so damage your sleep patterns and your capacity to concentrate
- You'll build better bone density, making osteoporosis much more unlikely (especially worth nothing if you are a female approaching or during the menopause)
- You will ease discomfort caused by rheumatism or generalised arthritis
- Your heart will work better (especially if you have had the misfortune to already have suffered any heart problems)

- Your digestive system will work much better
- If your blood pressure is raised, it will start to fall
- If you suffer low back pain, you will find it relieved
- You will sleep better

To strengthen your muscles as you do these exercises, your body releases those vital recovery hormones - yes, the ones that work overnight, using up extra fat. In those vital first four hours of Slow Wave Sleep, the exercises you have done during the day will be reaping you benefits.

Your body fat will be burning away as the hormones get on with their maintenance and repair; work, and your whole sense of wellbeing will be vastly improved as a result. You are not just burning fat, you're burning it for a benefit. So your skin, your internal organs, your teeth, hair and your bone mass are all improving while you sleep.

And here's the bonus-bonus. If you decide that you either don't want to or can't manage any specific resistance exercises, you will still benefit from the Hibernation Diet. You will have and notice the changes in how you look, feel and sleep. What exercising does is to add to these advantages.

The Birds and the Bees

We told you that we'd like you to understand a little bit more about the biology behind the Hibernation Diet, so here it comes. You won't need an 'A' level in science to understand it. It all hinges on how our brains need access to fuel during the night, and how taking honey before bed allows our bodies to burn fat while we sleep.

Honey is mankind's oldest sweetener.

Cave paintings in Spain from 7,000 years ago show scenes of men extracting honey from natural hives. Honey was used by the ancient Egyptians as a food and as a medicinal agent. The philosophers Plato and Aristotle make references to honey in their writings. The ancient Greek Olympic athletes used honey and figs as fuel for exercise and for sport.

To make one pound of honey bees must tap two million flowers for nectar and, from one hive, the bees will fly 55,000 miles to get it and bring it home. Honey bees can fly up to 22 miles per hour, and their fuel is so efficient that it is said that one bee could fly round the world on as little as an ounce of honey.

Bees are supremely intelligent little insects. An entomologist at the University of Montana, Jerry Bromenshenk, is training his bees to detect land mines. He conditions his bees with TNT dipped in syrup so that they can recognise the deadly explosive.

Honey is rich in nutrients and contains a great variety of vitamins, minerals, anti-oxidants and amino acids, the building blocks of proteins. Honey contains pyridoxine (vitamin B6), thiamine (vitamin B1), riboflavin (vitamin B2) and pantothenic acid (vitamin B5). Essential minerals include calcium, copper, iron, magnesium, manganese, phosphorous, potassium, sodium and zinc.

Honey has powerful anti-bacterial properties and research into its use for burns and post-surgery wound healing has confirmed this. Other conditions for which honey has shown promise include allergies and oral health.

But perhaps the most surprising thing of all about honey is that it actually lowers the glucose levels in your blood and that's been proved scientifically.

Honey has two kinds of sugar: glucose and fructose, in equal amounts, so you might expect it to raise blood glucose.

But here's the biological explanation. When sugars are absorbed from your gut into your bloodstream, they first go through your liver. It's here that the fructose is extracted. Only the liver can do that because only the liver has the enzyme to take fructose in.

In your liver the fructose is converted into glucose and then stored. It doesn't get passed back out into your bloodstream. It sits there until it's needed, which is when your blood glucose level falls.

And fructose has another clever ploy. It allows the liver to take in as much glucose as it needs out of the bloodstream, so that it can keep that greedy brain of yours properly fed. So the fructose is actually lowering the glucose levels in your bloodstream.

It sounds like a contradiction, which is why we have called it the fructose paradox. Because it involves glucose uptake by the liver, it stops a sudden rise in blood glucose. Fructose, if you like, lowers the Glycaemic Index (GI) of glucose, the speed at which food gets processed into blood glucose. It's a fabulous, wonderful trick to regulate blood glucose levels and it must have been one of nature's best-kept secrets until the Hibernation Diet came along.

Honey isn't the only place you'll find fructose, though it's the most concentrated source. It's also in fruit and vegetables in an equal balance with glucose. So the Hibernation Diet uses natural fructose to regulate blood glucose levels, keep the hungry brain fed, especially during the night, and does it without sudden peaks and troughs.

THE HUNGRY BRAIN

The brain is the greediest organ in the human body, and by a long distance. Keeping a good supply of glucose to it 24 hours a day is a big problem for us humans.

You know how exhausted you feel after concentrating for a long time. You think to yourself, 'But I've only been working at my desk! Why do I feel as if I'd run a marathon?' We're back to TATT here, because our brain is, of course, in constant use. It doesn't go to sleep when we do. It just keys down a bit.

The truth is that mental exhaustion is often greater than the physical kind, especially when it is ongoing. Even when it's resting, your brain burns up to 20 times more fuel than any other tissue in your body.

The trouble is that the brain is like a furnace in an old-fashioned steam engine. You have to shovel in fuel constantly to keep it going, and it can't store any of its own, so the possibility of stoking up the boiler and leaving it for a few hours isn't available. The fire would've gone out, and before it did, the engine would have pretty much ground to a halt and be incapable of doing anything useful. It burns intensely and constantly, so it has to be fuelled constantly.

It's your liver that stores and releases glucose around your body – and your brain grabs most of it. That's why keeping your liver's store of glycogen – the proper name for the energy it's storing – is so important. And honey is an easy, accessible, practical, efficient way of doing this.

If your blood glucose level drops, even by a small amount, your brain will panic. You start pumping out dangerously toxic amounts of hormones in a desperate effort to get more glucose up to your brain. They'll do their job, your brain will get the glucose released, but you'll suffer the after-effects if it happens frequently.

Too much of these hormones pulsing around your system and you're preparing the route to outcomes like heart disease, osteoporosis, obesity, Type 2 diabetes, poor immune system, depression, memory loss and a whole batch of other distressing conditions.

Make sure you've got your liver stored up properly by eating the right balance of carbohydrates from fructose/glucose sources and you will keep your brain happy. Keeping your brain fuelled means you don't need to pump out those dangerous hormones, so your body can get on with what you want it to do - burn up your extra fat during the night as fuel to rebuild your body.

How to Be a Hibernation Diet Expert

You will now have a pretty clear idea about what's going on in your body and how the Hibernation Diet makes the most of it. You'll know what to eat and when, why it will change your entire body recovery system and how much better you're going to feel.

You probably have some questions in your mind. Why should it work when everything else I have tried doesn't? What's so dramatically different here? How do I control my appetite?

These are the kinds of questions we'll answer in this section.

HUNGER: WHERE AND WHAT IS IT?

Have you ever asked yourself where you feel hungry? What is hunger and where does it come from? It's unlikely that anyone reading this book is physically starving. We have plenty of food around us, but how do we know when we're truly hungry and how do we manage it?

'I'm hungry. I've got a sort of pain in my stomach. I know I haven't eaten since breakfast'. That's hunger, plain and simple, isn't it?

But it isn't that simple, because hunger affects your head, liver, blood circulation, bones, arms and legs, muscles, even your heart.

Think about how hunger shows itself. Some people say they feel dizzy, shaking, sweating, confused, anxious, even aggressive. These are common side-effects of the human need for fuel.

It's difficult to pin it down. Different people will have different descriptions of how they feel.

So what? I mean, what's important is that my body is able to tell me it needs fuelled – not the detail of the how, where, what and why?

True up to a point, but the amorphous nature of hunger is interesting. We think of hunger as located in the stomach, and yet many of the reasons for it have little to do with the stomach itself and can be coming from locations quite a long way distant.

Hunger looks like some kind of global feeling of discomfort which is certainly manifest in the stomach but which reaches out to a number of other locations too.

It's a generalised feeling that seems to mutate around our bodies. We know there's a biological reason for it, yet we can't really pin it down so we're not sure how best to handle it.

Wait a minute. Is what you're saying that I ought to be able to identify which bit of my body is hungry at any one time?

In the Hibernation Diet we locate hunger in three distinct regions of the body, in the liver, in the brain and in the blood.

In the brain the hunger centre is located in the limbic region which is really your unconscious mind.

We aren't aware of the mammoth amount of work going on up there, but if it wasn't, we'd expire very quickly – in a matter of minutes.

Your liver is also processing away quietly in the background and it doesn't need any direct information from our mouths to work, but it's almost as vital as what's going on up in our brains.

All we're aware of is that if there's a lack of something, then we start to feel pretty strange. We can find ourselves unable to concentrate, suddenly very tired, unable to remember anything, feeling aggressive and irritable.

It's not only a matter of food but also those hormones that we don't pay much attention to, but which oil our human engines all the time. Without them, we'd crank to a stop.

Okay, I'll wear the idea of a hungry brain. That seems reasonable, but a hungry liver?

The liver is our energy and food warehouse, the storage, processing and distribution centre. It's where you can store a small amount of glycogen. It has to be kept replenished or your brain is in trouble.

Our bloodstream is the vehicle for delivering energy, nutrition, water and oxygen around our vital organs, and for getting rid of the waste through the kidneys and digestive system.

And it's on the liver that the brain depends entirely for its vital fuel. Though the liver is quite a big organ and richly supplied with blood, it can't hold very much brain fuel – only about 75–80g of glucose, enough for a few hours, so long as you aren't doing anything too strenuous.

We're using up the store at a furious rate just to keep our brains fed, and our kidneys and red blood cells are gobbling up glucose at a tremendous rate too.

So what happens if the liver runs out of fuel?

Fortunately, the brain thinks ahead. It doesn't wait until the liver is exhausted. It gets nervous feedback from the liver long before that stage, telling it how the glycogen level stands and how rapidly the fuel supply is being utilised.

As the level falls, and even while blood glucose is stable, the brain starts getting ready to cope with total depletion. To wait until there was no glycogen left would be suicidal.

Falling blood glucose (hypoglycaemia) is a warning of the catastrophe up ahead, and at this point the brain is close to meltdown.

Now we'll start pumping out those dangerous hormones, adrenaline and cortisone, and it's their job to release any leftovers of glucose they can find.

But why's that dangerous? Surely that's a good thing?

You'd think so, and it is in a way because if they didn't go out, that'd be it. The trouble is that they are emergency services. They go wherever they have to as quickly as possible to get that glucose. And where do they go? Off to the muscles which are then degraded to give the liver glucose again.

All the non-essential functions get shut down. Things like your gut and immune system go off message. Your muscles are under attack now. Cortisone also degrades your bones, so this hormone army won't be seen as rescuers there.

Your heart rate speeds up and your blood pressure rises. You may get sweaty and start shaking. You can't think straight and your speech may be slurred or muddled.

So where's the hunger thing then?

Now that we've got a fuller picture of what's going on inside, we can see that it has to be the liver that sends out the first critical 'feed me!' message. But it's not out to feed itself alone. It's out to feed everything from our brains to our toenails. That's why you need to understand a little of what's going on in your body.

Because the Hibernation Diet matches your fuel needs to foods that will make you feel satisfied, not hungry, you'll find yourself much more aware of the messages that say 'I want to eat!' and be able to provide the best kinds of food to meet the need. You'll find that you will feel hungry much less frequently as a result of taking in the right kind of fuel mix, so you won't want to nibble and graze on fast foods or sugary drinks.

REAL LIFE: JACKIE'S HELPFUL HORMONES

Jackie is 21, and she enjoys the running she mostly does alongside her pal, Caroline, but last year she was in the pits of despair.'I'd been training for the London Marathon. I'm what you'd call a "recreational" runner. I'm not a sports or fitness junkie, but I do like running, and Caroline and I go out maybe two or three times a week, sometimes more.

'I really, really wanted to do the London Marathon. It was a big deal for me, to see if I could keep going that long, but I was a bit chunky then, probably about six pounds heavier than I should've been.

'It seemed to become a big rubicon, something I had to cross. Everyone seemed to be going on at me about it, from the trainer we had to help us - there were nine of us aiming for the Marathon to raise money for Diabetes – to my own mum!

'The trainer said I just had to "eat less and lose the lard," as he put it, but I couldn't shift it, no matter what I did. I trained more, I cut down on carbohydrates, and all I felt was worse and the same size. It hit my confidence, and the

Marathon looked like a non-starter for me.

'To be honest, the Hibernation Diet seemed ridiculous. They were telling me to increase my carbohydrate intake. There was a lot of stuff about liver function and doing less running. I thought they were mad. It was the opposite of what the trainer was telling me to do.

'But you reach a point where you'll try anything, and I thought, why not give it a go? I did see the biological sense behind it once it was explained, and the idea that you could be using the extra food you ate to burn up weight at night was so novel it had to be true. No one could have made that up.

'That's where the hormones came in. The extra calories would mobilise hormones that would break down and use fat – those recovery hormones – especially at night.

'I started to feed up my liver with fresh and dried fruit and honey before bed. I cut back on low-level aerobic exercise and worked on shorter periods of resistance-based exercise.

'And the proof of the pudding? I lost the fat, felt stronger and fitter, and I beat Caroline in the London Marathon.'

FAT: WHERE AND WHAT IS IT?

Now we know a bit more about hunger, what about fat? What is it that actually makes us eat too much and get too fat in the first place? You can meet two people with very similar eating habits, same age, gender, lifestyle, and yet one can be really obese while the other is slim and lithe.

What's behind all this? Is it our metabolism? Is it our anxiety level? Or is it less about the amount of food we eat and rather more about our food choices?

Here are some of the answers that show why the Hibernation Diet is far more than a diet.

Look, we've all been looking for the ultimate diet pill that evaporates fat or burns calories. The nearest we've got is horror stomach-stapling and liposuction. So this notion of burning fat up while you sleep is daft.

We love instant solutions. A new fad diet, a new pill, the promise of eternal youth, and we're out there, queuing up to spend our hard-earned cash on drugs that interfere with what our bodies want to do. Then we wonder why we suffer from side-effects.

We're showing you how to use your body's biology to your own advantage. know you can burn more calories at night than you're doing now and we know how to do it.

It'll work because, in fact, it can't fail. You aren't putting anything weird in. You aren't extracting anything out. You are simply exploiting what's already there. The only reason it could fail would be if your liver wasn't storing glycogen, if your brain didn't need food and if your lovely helpful hormones decided to go on strike and not do any of that repair work, and if that were the case, you wouldn't actually be here reading this.

But still, isn't the case that there will always been some people who get fat and others who don't?

Yes, we all have to live with our DNA and its individual mix of the desirable and undesirable. The fact that every single one of us has a unique DNA that shows in everything from a hair to a heart is one good reason why there's no 'one cure for all' when it comes to weight loss.

The basics are the same: eat more than you burn and you'll put on weight, just as the opposite is equally true: eat less than you burn and you'll lose it. But while some people struggle against gaining weight all their lives, others seem to be able to eat whatever they like and maintain a stable, healthy, svelte figure.

Each one of us has something we'll call a Metabolic Personality (MP) all our own. It's made up of our genes, the environment and lifestyle we live with, how we've been brought up, our attitudes to food and exercise, even the weather, and a host of other variables.

Even though there's an average number of calories we each need to keep the main functions like our heart, digestion, brain activity and circulation going, there's still a lot of room for differences within that average.

A host of hormones influence when each of us feels hungry or thirsty. As we eat and digest, other signals come into play telling our brains what's needed to keep us alert and functioning normally.

The way these hormones are released is in turn altered by factors like exercise, the menstrual cycle, tiredness, even a virus like flu.

For some of us, a regular exercise routine will work wonders, while another person says it makes no difference. Some of us seem to build muscle and get rid of excess fat easily, while others pound it out in the gym for no visible results at all.

Success or failure plays into our mental attitude and our self-belief, and that in turn impacts on how we look and feel about ourselves. It alters our emotions too. We're familiar with comfort eating and the problems of anorexia and bulimia that, according to some estimates, probably affect something like one in ten of us.

The way forward is not to look for solutions from bottles and fad diets, but to use our own uniquely individual metabolic personality to manage appetite and enjoy a stable, healthy weight.

But how do I know what my Metabolic Personality is?

WHY YOUR METABOLIC PERSONALITY MATTERS

You would like to weigh less. You're advised to cut calories but it isn't working. Everyone has a different metabolic personality, and the variation between two people could be as much as 300 per cent. Even two sisters, eating similar food and living similar lifestyles, could have very different outcomes on the same calorie-reduced diet. What makes the difference? Your body manages your weight using hormones, glands and your nervous system to manage the fuel balance. There's a whole myriad of complex pathways for the information to travel around your liver, heart, digestive system, brain, blood and vital other essential functions. What you eat and how hungry you are form just the tip of a food and energy iceberg. It's your metabolic personality that dictates the terms.

HIBERNATION DIET METABOLIC PERSONALITIES

The Hibernation Diet has identified four different metabolic personalities:

Type HD1

These are the fast movers with a fast metabolism. They're the driven types, highly focused and dynamic, often workaholics and usually highly successful in whatever is their chosen field. They drive their families, friends and colleagues to distraction because they never seem to be able to turn off and chill out. As a result, they place enormous demands upon their bodies and make themselves vulnerable to heart attacks and other stress-related serious medical conditions. They seldom become overweight, but because life in the fast lane means constantly pumping out stress hormones, they pay a high price in overall health and wellbeing. Their capacity to benefit from overnight recovery is drastically reduced from its potential. Because they produce so much adrenaline and cortisone, their poor livers have to search constantly for new fuel supplies, keeping their bodies in a near-constant state of panic.

Type HD2

These are the people at the other end of the extreme, the genuinely slow metabolisers. This type of metabolic personality is very efficient. In fact, it's so efficient that its owners tend to get fat because their bodies are so good at drawing out every gram of goodness from their food. Their digestive systems take their time about doing this, so there's plenty of scope to build up good fat stores. This one is the Eskimo, the one who tends to lay down lots of cosy layers to keep him or herself safe during the long, cold winter. This is the real hibernation animal and these folk survive famine brilliantly, their brains and livers drawing on all that goodness stored away as fat. To add to their difficulties, they get told that a slow metabolism is just a myth and being overweight is all their own fault. But it isn't true. A metabolic specialist from Arizona, Eric Ravussin, proved beyond any doubt that our basic metabolic rate can vary anywhere between usage of about 1,000 calories a day up to 3,000.

Type HD3

These are life's fidgets, the people who can sit all right but never sit quite still. They're the ones that the teacher used to yell at; 'James, will you for heaven's sake stop fidgeting!' But for James, and all the others like him, all that moving around requires quite a lot of energy output.

Since it's happening when the body is generally at rest, the muscles are using only fat to provide the 'fidget calories'. That means all the energy that fidgets use up while they're technically sitting is coming out of their fat stores. And if you fidget all day every day, then the effect can be very significant. On top of that, if you're a daytime fidget, you're probably a night one as well, so you get an additional bonus when you're asleep. If you're interested, it was a smart guy called James A. Levine at the Mayo Clinic in the US who worked this one out.

Type HD4

If you're unfortunate enough to fall into this category, it can be a real trial to get excess weight off. These are the people who just don't respond to exercise. No one really understands why this is, although there's a lot of research going on. One person can do three short sessions of exercise a week and see the weight falling off during those crucial Slow Wave Sleep hours, while the HD4s watch enviously, do as much or more work, and just don't see any effects at all. But don't despair. Even if your body has some secret trick that enables you to protect all your fat stores to the bitter end, the Hibernation Diet will work for you because you *aren't* exercising during the night. Besides, you're the people in the gene pool with the best survival rates, and you're cuddly!

You may well have already been able to recognise your type here, but take this quiz to refine your ideas. Give yourself one point for each 'yes' in each of the two columns. Only tick the statements that are right for you.

Test yourself

1 FAST METABOLISERS: HD1 AND HD3

1. I am strong and muscular with a powerful body
2. My ears look darker than the rest of my face
3. My eyes are very moist and sometimes tears appear for no reason
4. The skin on my face is bright, radiant and shiny
5. My skin tends to be oily and quite highly coloured
6. I get a runny nose quite a lot
7. My nails are thin and bend easily
8. I often get itches, especially on my scalp, arms or calves
9. My weight gain tends to be on my upper body
10. I don't like too much heat
11. I get a strong reaction to insect bites and stings, with swelling and pain, itching, bruising, redness
12. Sometimes I'll get a sneezing attack, even though I don't have a cold
13. I drive myself hard in every area and am ambitious
14. I can be too short-tempered and anxious
15. I'm good at multi-tasking
16. I'm very socially outgoing and love good company
17. I love to eat. It's a big part of my life
18. I don't sleep well unless I've had something to eat before bedtime
19. Skipping a meal makes me feel cross and tired
20. Sometimes I eat far more than I know I need
21. I gag very easily. A sudden bad smell always makes me throw up
22. I don't really suffer from unexpected thirst, though I love salty foods
23. I like strongly sharp foods like pickles, citrus fruit, sauerkraut, lemons, yoghurt
24. I enjoy fatty foods more than sweet ones
25. Coffee makes me feel jittery, nervous, even sick

Total for Column 1 [　]

2. SLOW METABOLISERS: HD2 AND HD4

1. My body shape is naturally curvy or pear-shaped with my strength concentrated around my hips and legs
2. My ears look pale against the rest of my face
3. My eyes are dry but don't tend to itch
4. My complexion tends to sallow and pale and rather dull or chalky
5. My nose is often too dry
6. I have tough fingernails, strong and hard
7. I very rarely suffer any kind of skin itch
8. Extra weight will tend to gather around my abdomen
9. I often feel cold and am happiest in warm weather and warm places
10. Insect bites don't tend to bother me much and go away quickly
11. It takes a lot to make me gag
12. I don't really sneeze unless I actually have a cold (or a specific allergy)
13. I'm very laid-back and even-tempered, hard to annoy
14. I'm rather subject to depression and a feeling of apathy or exhaustion
15. I approach problems one by one rather than try to multi-task
16. I feel very uncomfortable at social gatherings and would rather be alone
17. I'm not very interested in food or cooking
18. I generally sleep soundly
19. If I skip a meal, it doesn't seem to make me feel bad
20. I almost never eat snacks
21. I get thirsty easily, though I don't eat much salt
22. I don't really like very sweet or very sour foods
23. I can easily go more than four hours without eating anything
24. I hate fatty foods
25. My morning coffee gives me a good start to the day

Total for Column 2 [　]

To work out your Metabolic Personality percentage

Add up the column scores separately, subtract the lower column result from the higher one. Now divide that figure by the number of statements you ticked and multiply it by 100 per cent.

Example: Vicky ticks 10 statements in Column 1 and 15 in Column 2. She subtracts 10 from 15 leaving 5. She divides five by 25 giving 0.2 and multiplies by 100 giving her 20. Vicky's metabolic personality puts her on the slow side of moderate.

My score for
Column 1 is:

My score for
Column 2 is:

Divide by statements ticked:

Multiply by 100:

**My final metabolic
score is:**

_____

A score of around 33 per cent indicates an average metabolism. A higher result will indicate that you are in the faster or slower regions according to which column dominates. You will be able to assess for yourself whether you have a tendency towards type **HD2 or HB4** from your personal score.

How to Achieve a Sense of Wellbeing

We all have a general sense of how our minds are affected by how we look. At one level, you know you feel great in a particular outfit, and that there are certain colours and styles that suit or don't suit you.

But your understanding of the Hibernation Diet will do far more than this.

As we've already made clear, your mental health can't be completely separated from your physical wellbeing, but it is difficult to follow the ways in which mental and physical health are interlinked.

Let's take a look at how what we eat, the exercise we take and our energy levels are linked together in the Hibernation Diet so as to provide the components of a balanced, healthy lifestyle that not only sees you slim and fit but also much more mentally and emotionally balanced than you may be feeling at the moment.

FOOD AND STRESS

Stress is all around us. We have to live with it, but there's a great deal we can do to minimise its grip. What we eat is a good starting point.

Too much chocolate can leave you feeling very weary once the short sugar and caffeine burst dies away. An overdose of salty crisps dehydrates your body and your brain, causing fatigue. High-fat meals raise your stress hormone levels and keep them high.

The trouble is we tend to reach out for exactly these kinds of foods at the worst possible times. They're quick, easy, available, and we train our bodies to crave them.

So when we feel dog-tired at work, anxious about something in our lives, we reach for the fast fix and we suffer the consequences.

Certain foods have brutal effects on the brain. Nutritional research has identified the foods that create stress and the ones that help to eliminate it. In a trial carried out by The Food and Mood Project, nearly 90 per cent of the 200 people in the sample reported that their mental health had improved significantly with changes in diet that they had made.

The Hibernation Diet uses that information so that you can avoid the 'food stressors' like sugar, caffeine, alcohol and chocolate. Our eating plan reaches for the advantageous food supporters like honey of course, water, vegetables, fruit and oil-rich fish.

And as well as what you eat, there's the critical factor of when you eat. Again, the Hibernation Diet tells you to eat frequently from healthy food choices, carrying nutritious snacks with you and planning your meals in advance.

We know already that stress hormones like cortisone rob our bodies of the vitamins they need, hijacking them to support all those classic symptoms of stress like the tensing up of muscles and rising blood pressure – reactions that are so important to that basic human 'fight or flight' response.

So when anxiety levels rise, we're especially in need of the B complex vitamins which help to maintain our nerves and brain cells. B vitamins are also used to convert food into energy in the body.

Which takes us back to that issue of how important it is to eat the right foods to respond to stress and anxiety. You might feel you want a packet of crisps, a tin of fizzy cola and a bar of chocolate, but what you're doing is adding to your body's strife. Even just a few days of vitamin B deficiency – maybe while you were especially under pressure at work – can cause mental havoc, upsetting the nervous system and compounding the stress. It's a classic double whammy.

Reach instead for something like a banana. For a meal, look towards baked potatoes, avocados, organic chicken and dark green leafy vegetables. They're loaded with B vitamins.

The more extreme the stress, the more dangerous the outcome of responding to it in the wrong way. As the stress hormones step up production, something like 1,400 chemical changes take place in our bodies, sapping us of vital nutrients including those B vitamins, vitamin C, vitamin A and the mineral, magnesium.

These hormones that are being pumped out also lower the level of serotonin, making us reach for instant carbs when in fact, if we reached instead for high fibre, low GI carbs, we'd do ourselves a big favour.

Reach for the instant solution – hamburger and chips, takeaway meals, white bread – and we're also setting ourselves up for weight gain and a much higher risk of heart disease.

When you're under pressure, you may well be contending with deadlines as well, so the temptation to reach for junk food is enormous. But stick with the Hibernation Diet food regime and you will truly feel the rewards.

EXERCISE AND STRESS

Aerobic exercise – anything that makes you feel breathless and hot – makes your heart work harder, your blood pump more, and can certainly reduce the risk of developing heart disease as well as helping you stay generally fit and trim.

We've already explained that resistance exercise works in a different way. If you can combine a mixture of the two kinds of exercise, you'll be complementing the Hibernation Diet process of overnight recovery and general fitness.

But you don't need to go for 10-mile runs or cycle up the side of a mountain. There's a growing body of evidence that shows that even as little as 10 minutes of resistance work a day can bolster your mental health and leave you thinking more clearly, feeling happier and less stressed. Add in 10 minutes of brisk walking, a swim or a cycle ride, and the effect will be even more dramatic.

Here are some of the direct ways in which exercise will help your mental health:

Exercise boosts your brain power

Providing that you keep your liver properly fuelled, exercise will help to pump blood around your system and improve its flow to your brain. You'll see faster reactions, better concentration, higher creativity and mental vigour as a result.

Exercise slows down mental ageing

In a recent study, researchers discovered that just walking regularly helped to prevent mental slowdown in women over the age of 65. The longer and more often they walked, the better was their mental sharpness. Best of all, most people start reaping these benefits after just a couple of months of three-times-a-week exercising, even though it wasn't intense.

Exercise with good recovery stops stress in its tracks

Exercise is a great way of reducing anxiety. You literally 'work it off', whatever kind of exercise you do. In resistance work, you find that your worries give way to concentration, and that in turn makes you feel more relaxed. The process of tensing and releasing your muscles lowers stress hormones and aids your night-time recovery at the same time. Meditative exercise such as yoga also helps you to centre yourself and creates a sense of calm.

Exercise gives you a natural high

Any kind of exercise will boost the levels of 'feel good' brain chemicals such as serotonin, dopamine and endorphins, the body's own painkillers.

A study in England found that 83 per cent of people with mental health problems relied on exercising to improve their mood and reduce anxiety. Anyone suffering from mild or moderate depression will benefit from regular exercise within 16 weeks and find that the impact is every bit as effective as taking prescribed anti-depressants such as Seroxat and Prozac, while avoiding all the downsides of drugs.

Exercise improves your sex life. Yes, it really does. Not just because you feel physically fitter and more attractive, but also because it releases hormones that impact upon your capacity to enjoy sex. Also, many people taking prescribed anti-depressants find themselves impotent and unable to enjoy sex. Much better to use Hibernation Diet principles and stick to exploiting your own internal resources.

Exercise flushes out toxins

Exercise is the most effective way of ridding your body of the build-up of stress, poor diet and perhaps too much alcohol. It acts as a natural anti-toxin, cleansing your system of the negative impact of a less than ideal lifestyle.

Exercise improves your sleep pattern

And we know how important sleep is. Exercising will mean you spend less of your sleeping hours in the REM (rapid eye movement) part of your sleep. Instead, you will spend more time in the Slow Wave Sleep cycle when your body is busy using up its fat stores in maintenance and repair. In REM sleep, you stop producing serotonin too, so opening the door to feeling depressed.

Exercise boosts your self-esteem

Getting stronger, leaner and fitter has a very positive effect upon how you feel about yourself. One recent study sampled teenagers who are active in sports and those who aren't. The active group had much better self-esteem than the 'couch potatoes'.

Exercise cuts back on the need to produce dangerous hormones.

The Hibernation Diet is focused upon ways of cutting back on the body's desire to pump them out. That means reducing output of cortisone from the adrenal glands around the neurones. When you get a major shock of any kind, cortisone dumps glucose from surrounding cells into brain cells and this is why we remember these painful events. The memory lives on because of the extra fuel available to the cell at the time.

We do need our cortisone production in times of real

crisis but when it is released on an ongoing level because of inadequate liver fuelling, it starts to destroy the brain cells. Too many attacks of low glucose levels in the blood lead to loss of cognitive function, so your memory begins to fail and you take much longer to respond to stimuli of any kind.

Too much cortisone production destroys brain cells, big time. We now know for definite that depression is closely linked to an excess of cortisone.

And by now you will know well how to avoid over-production of cortisone and the other dangerous adrenal hormones: keep that liver properly fuelled!

We all want to feel good. The irony is that we literally have it within our own power to make sure that we do. Yes, there will be crises in all our lives, difficult and painful traumas to weather, but we can do a great deal to help ourselves deal with it and come through it if we listen closely to our own internal needs.

DEPRESSION AND WEIGHT GAIN

'Fat and happy' used to be a popular myth. Do you know anyone who is happy to be fat? There's a direct connection here between weight gain and depression and it's focused on the adrenal glands. It's a classic Catch-22. Each problem contributes to and is being caused by the other one. When you try to resolve the outcome, you recreate the conditions that brought it about in the first place.

So let's take a closer look at the links between weight gain and mild to moderate depression.

Do you suffer from any of these problems?

- Low self-esteem
- Poor motivation levels
- Lethargy/weariness

- Apathy
- Bursts of uncontrollable crying
- Panic attacks
- Poor concentration
- Memory loss
- A sense of mental exhaustion
- Poor appetite
- Digestive problems
- Repeated bouts of colds and flu
- Loss of libido
- Weight gain
- Disrupted menstrual cycle
- Frequent headaches
- Overheating and sweats
- Insomnia

All these can be symptoms of what's known as sub-clinical depression. That is, the opening pointers to depression before it has reached the level at which you may decide the only solution is prescribed anti-depressant drugs.

Ever since the 1950s depression has been growing towards epidemic levels. In the last fifty years or so there's been a huge increase in highly processed fast food. We're eating it on the run, we're drowning our bodies in saturated fat, and we're feeling tired and enervated. We try to escape through the worst possible routes: a shot of caffeine, a long drink of fizzy coke full of nothing but sugar, colourings and a lot of unpronounceable additives.

The debilitating effects of this and of stress-related conditions such as anxiety, sleeplessness, sudden mood swings and panic attacks can be treated through the Hibernation Diet approach to healthy living and exercise because they all relate directly to over production of adrenal hormones – better known as stress hormones.

In the past, when maintaining regular supplies of food was critical, weight gain was seen as a measure of success and was certainly not viewed as something negative. We see this in the art of ancient cultures: the symbol of optimum health was a well-rounded, amply fertile, female figure.

Now excess weight is regarded as taboo, both generally and in the body-conscious media. Overweight people feel like social outcasts.

The thinking part of our brains, the bit at the top, the cortex, may feel uncomfortable about being overweight, but the body 'thinks' differently. The connecting system between mind and body is the central emotional (limbic) system, which regulates interchanges between the two regions. If we think negatively about our body image, the emotional system will regulate the production of hormones to reflect this and there will be ongoing negative effects on the body.

If we go to a film or to a play which is sad, then our immune system takes an instant dive. We suddenly become more vulnerable to infections. Why? That external unhappiness creates a reaction in our internal emotional system and we start pumping out adrenal hormones. The hormone most directly linked to suppression of the immune system is cortisone. So, yes, depression does make you ill.

The pituitary gland activates the adrenal glands when we're stressed, but it also regulates production of the wonderful recovery hormones.

Is there, therefore, a connection to be made between weight gain and depression? Most definitely, and it is quite independent of the question of social rejection.

A trial of patients taking the SSRI anti-depressants like Prozac and Seroxat showed that a side-effect was often weight loss, especially early in the treatment. It wasn't necessarily maintained, but the effect was quite clear and gave the research teams a real puzzle.

Why should this be? Why would anti-depressants have such an impact on weight?

The answer is cortisone production. Cortisone makes us gain weight because it promotes another hormone, properly called NPY and nicknamed by the Hibernation Diet as HCH – the hamburger-and-chip hormone.

We head for a fast food outlet, eat the biggest cheeseburger we can buy and drink a couple of litres of cola. The cheeseburger gives us a huge splurge of saturated fats which are quickly stored in our various fat-storing regions. The massive sugar load has to be dealt with quickly before the glucose jamming up our blood vessels causes irreversible damage. The pancreas pumps out tidal waves of insulin. The blood glucose falls rapidly. Any sugar finding its way into the liver is converted to fat.

Now there is no glucose left in the liver to re-supply the blood and brain. The brain panics, causes cortisone release from the adrenals, driving up production of HCH, and we are very quickly driven back to junk food, hungry for more of the same. It's a vicious circle and the only beneficiaries are the hamburger sellers.

Junk food gives a sudden blood glucose rise. That kicks in insulin production to bring it down and that's then followed by another urgent craving and upsurge in cortisone production, while we crave more fast carbs to get the blood glucose up again, which pushes out insulin again...and so it continues.

Not only does cortisone production impact on weight, but it is a recognised component in depression.

For several decades depression was associated with low levels of serotonin in the brain. This theory is now fast becoming redundant and, although serotonin is involved, we now know that the key hormone of depression is cortisone.

Cortisone regulates energy levels in the brain. Cortisone is released whenever the liver store is depleted, when blood glucose is in danger of falling and the brain will run out of energy. A rapid release of cortisone provides increased energy from the liver store, but if the store is already low, then more and more cortisone needs to be released and this gets in the way of delivering energy to the brain.

An emergency release of cortisone in a real 'fight or flight' situation is good. Chronic production of it is not. It's when this happens that cortisone plays havoc in the brain, destroying cells in key regions. What is beneficial in certain situations becomes thoroughly damaging. In its wake, all this non-emergency cortisone production leads to depression.

It's rather like keeping the sirens wailing and the lights flashing on an ambulance when there's no one in it. The idea of an emergency becomes redundant but the lights and noise go on anyway.

The SSRIs and other anti-depressive drugs act on weight regulation by countering the damage to the brain caused by chronic over-production of cortisone by the adrenal glands.

Modern processed and refined foods result in continual liver fuel shortages, undermine blood glucose stability, threaten energy supply to the hungry brain which then panics and activates the adrenal stress glands, leading to chronic over-production of cortisone.

Just after a mother gives birth, she's often quite euphoric and bursting with delight, but some suffer from severe depression at this stage, sometimes so bad that they are unable to bond with their babies or even care very much what happens to them.

The difference?

The euphoric mothers have very low levels of cortisone, while the depressed mothers have very high levels.

It's a very different situation from depression caused by a fast food diet, but the effect is similar. In the case of postnatal depression, the impact of massive changes in levels of fertility hormones is responsible, but the importance of keeping cortisone production under control is evident for both groups of people.

There is one last little twist in this junk food revolving-door syndrome. An empty liver, a hungry brain and too much cortisone have another dangerous effect: cortisone breaks down muscle and bone in its desperate search for fuel to give to the liver.

The liver enzymes, the busy workers who perform the task of turning that fuel around and getting it off to the brain, turn out in force. Too much force to be good for us.

The Hibernation Diet provides the healthy way forward, the right way to calm your adrenals by making sure your liver is properly fed with the fructose it can use to keep your brain happy – and fight off depression in the process.

Tired All the Time?

We spoke of TATT early on, but now we'd like to explore this cry for help a little more. We aren't talking here about the kind of physical tiredness you get after a long hike, but about that sense of general weariness that bedevils so many of us.

TATT is a wretched but totally avoidable state – a direct and inevitable consequence of the modern diet. Its highly refined carbohydrates and sugars just don't give our brains that continuous supply of essential glucose that is so vital. Instead, we convert these fast-food sugars into fats and store them around our bodies. To change it, we need to look closely at the kinds of foods we eat and we need to have an understanding of why they're the wrong fuel for our internal furnace.

If you put petrol into a diesel engine car, you destroy it, and the cost of cleaning out the system is massive. If you don't expect a diesel engine to run on petrol, why should you expect your biological furnace to work off fast food and highly refined carbs?

Ask yourself these questions:

- Do you wake up exhausted in the early hours of the morning?
- Do you find it difficult to sleep?

- Is your weight hard to control?
- Do you get hunger pangs all the time?
- Do you crave sweet food?
- Do you feel exhausted after a meal?
- Do you get drowsy spells during the day?
- Do you find your thinking gets muddled?
- Do you have a poor memory?
- Do you get inexplicable mood swings?

If we go back to around the end of the nineteenth century, we find doctors focusing on fatigue. They saw it as 'central' fatigue, coming from the brain and were worried that students could be overburdened with their studies, which could lead to a host of medical and psychological problems.

They were well ahead of their time. The epidemic of mental and physical breakdowns we see today was being predicted in their writing and research work.

In the twentieth century, research turned towards developing drugs to solve all our health problems. Rather than looking inside the human body, science shifted towards looking for off-the-clinical-shelf remedies to cure everything from obesity to schizophrenia.

It has taken over 100 years for the research to come full circle.

Fatigue causes stress; stress causes fatigue. The two are mutually intertwined in the debilitating and toxic cycle now so common in western society.

If you recognised your own symptoms in three or more of the questions, then you are indeed TATT. You are chronically fatigued. This, by the way, is not to say that you are suffering from the particular condition known as ME, or Chronic Fatigue Syndrome, a particular type of illness requiring specialist treatment.

You are, though, living with a feeling of constant exhaustion and weariness that is a result of how your liver is struggling to cope with the demands of your brain, and how you are flooding yourself with dangerous hormones to try to make up the shortfall.

Think of a difficult day at work, a day full of stresses of one kind or another, a frustrating day, when you felt you didn't really achieve anything. You came home, had a go at the children and snapped at your mother on the phone. Even driving home was a nightmare. You felt so tired that all you wanted to do was sink into the sofa and sleep.

You probably hardly got up from your desk. You sat in front of your computer struggling with the latest crises, grabbed a snack pizza at lunchtime and tanked up with several cups of coffee. You felt sleepy and exhausted all day, yet you had done nothing more physical that turn your computer on.

You just didn't have the energy to cook a sensible meal, so you satisfied your pangs with a couple of packets of crisps and a drink of fizzy lemonade. Once the children were asleep, you went to bed for the night, more weary than if you had run a marathon.

You spent a restless and uncomfortable night, feeling hot and sweaty, dozing then waking up every 15 minutes When you woke at about three o'clock, you felt hungry but too weary to do anything about it.

When you finally got up in the morning, you felt at least as tired as when you went to bed, which in turn made you feel downright miserable and tearful as you faced another day of stressful trials at home and at work.

Why? You hadn't done anything physical. Your day at work was no worse and no better than usual. The children weren't especially irritating and the traffic no more chaotic than ever.

As a matter of fact, you will indeed get up fatter, heavier, slower, weaker, sicker and more fatigued than when you went to bed.

WEIGHING IT ALL UP

Take Kerry. She was asking herself this question.

'I am carrying around 10 kilos of fat more than I need or want. That's 10,000 grams of fat and fat has some nine calories to the gram.

'So I have 90,000 calories extra for my body to use to give me some energy during the day and for recovery overnight.

'Why, in the midst of this plenty, am I so constantly tired and drained, lacking in any motivation and feeling irritable and unhappy?

'I have all this spare energy but I can't seem to use it.

'I know tiredness is central and that the brain needs constant feeding. I know it'll want about 600 calories every 24 hours, but hasn't it got 90,000 of them at its disposal?

'I mean, if I had £90,000 and I spent £600 on a holiday, it'd hardly deplete my reserves, would it? That's only about 0.6 per cent of my fund!'

Trouble is, of course, to take the economic metaphor a bit further, the currency conversion. There isn't one. It would be a little like trying to take your old Italian Lire into the bank to get Euros. The two have been separated and the first no longer has any currency.

It isn't convertible.

None of these spare calories can be turned into the glucose Kerry's brain demands. Not *one* of all the calories contained in this massive energy reserve can be taken up so productively. The Lire – and Kerry's excess fat – are no use in this state.

Calories stored as fat are used for two purposes only: as a back-up fuel reserve during exercise and as fuel to provide the energy for the night-time recovery that lies at the very centre of the Hibernation Diet.

Following the Hibernation Diet allows your body to

access those fat reserves constructively during the night, burning them up for your benefit.

Think of it this way. If it was possible to convert our fat stores into glucose for the brain, nobody on the planet would need to be obese. The greedy and sweet-toothed brain would simply burn up our spare fat every minute of every hour for 24 hours of every day. Obesity could not exist.

The downside would be that we'd have no reserve to fall back on when there was a shortage of food, or a marathon run in the offing. Evolution wouldn't have been able to cope with that and the human species would have perished long ago.

So central fatigue is a dangerous condition where the brain is constantly deprived of a stable energy store because, although there are massive quantities of energy potentially available, they cannot be accessed.

All that reserve is sitting there, yet our brains are being starved of the fuel they need and our livers aren't able to supply it. We get low blood glucose levels that lead to headaches, irritability, lack of concentration, inability to focus, and start us pumping out those dangerous hormones again, bringing on more unpleasant side effects.

The Hibernation Diet solution

So let's take a look at what Kerry eats on an average day.

She gets up at 7.30 in the morning, dashes around in a frenzy getting the kids sorted and out to school. She grabs a cup of coffee. At about 11 o'clock, she usually has another coffee and a chocolate biscuit bar.

Lunchtime varies and can be anywhere between 12 and, well, not at all. Sometimes she'll grab a sandwich and eat it at her desk. It's usually of white bread and filled with either bacon, lettuce and tomato or prawn mayonnaise. Sometimes she'll get a hamburger and a fizzy drink instead. If she has errands to do, she'll probably just skip lunch altogether.

In the middle of the afternoon, Kerry feels tired and ravenous. She'll tuck into the communal biscuit tin in the office and have one or two more cups of coffee.

By the time she gets home at around 6.30 in the evening, she's exhausted and irritable. The kids have to be fed and she's careful to make sure they eat well, but for herself, she'll finish off their leftovers and flop on to the sofa with a glass of wine.

About eight, she gets the children to bed, watches TV for a while then sorts out domestic chores like washing and ironing before she takes herself off to bed.

What Kerry needs to do

Kerry needs to tackle the causes of her constant tiredness. There are eight crucial times of the day where she needs to take particular action:

Early morning: Kerry wakes up feeling wretched because she hasn't fed her liver before bed. It has spent the night using up muscle to keep Kerry's brain in business. The liver has been denied the opportunity to go and use calories out of fat stores for recovery because it's been in panic mode trying to find brain fuel from wherever it can – by degrading muscle. As well as that, the absence of decent liver fuel means that Kerry won't have been able to get the repair and maintenance teams out to rebuild bone, cell and tissue, so she's going to get up feeling really tired.

Cure factor: Before Kerry begins to tackle her diet generally, she needs to start getting at least a tablespoon of honey into her system an hour or so before bed. She could very usefully make it into a drink that she would enjoy and which would provide her with a host of other nutrients as well. At breakfast time, she absolutely must make time for herself and select a breakfast from the Hibernation Diet plan. Her system is screaming for fructose sources that it can bring to the liver so as to be ready to take on the day.

Mid-morning: Already, Kerry will be feeling more in control than ever before. She will find her concentration level much better and she won't keep forgetting important matters at work.

Cure factor: To reinforce this, she needs to forgo the coffee and exchange it for a fruit or herbal tea or a long drink of water along with a piece of fruit or a small handful of nuts and seeds.

After lunch: Kerry's after-lunch weariness comes from her choice of high GI (glycaemic index) food sources. The highly refined ingredients in burgers and white bread give her a blood glucose surge that then falls again very quickly as it's hit with insulin. She needs to eat something that will stabilise her blood glucose level and provide nutrition for a few hours.

Cure factor: Dump the junk and have a decent, organic wholemeal bread sandwich made at home or at work from her own choice of ingredients. There are plenty of alternatives in the Hibernation Diet menu plans. It's important at this time of day that Kerry tops up on the fructose so that she prevents a post lunch blood glucose crash and the hormone production that follows on. Fructose now will also provide Kerry with a good metabolic environment for optimum performance as the working day goes on.

Later in the afternoon: Because her system hasn't been fed the right fuel, Kerry has been topping up her starving liver with sweet biscuits and coffee.

Cure factor: What Kerry needs to do is to take the longer view, providing the right kind of fuel for her internal engine and avoiding the fat storage that follows on from high GI food intake. She should look to a cereal bar for example, or pick an alternative from the diet plans.

Going home: At the moment, Kerry finds going home a terrible trial. She doesn't feel able to cope with the traffic; she's tired and anxious and irritable. She does keep a packet or two of crisps in the car and sometimes eats some while she drives.

Cure factor: There's often an energy crash towards the end of the working day. It's caused by a mix of the emotional 'end of the day' factors and food resources, but Kerry can avoid being pitched into it very simply. Ditch the crisps and have a small bottle of fresh fruit juice instead. She will find herself a lot less stressed when she drives and will be able to shake off that irritability.

Dinner time and into the evening: Kerry's life has a lot of stress factors: her job, travelling and of course the children, of which she has two, aged 11 and seven. She's a great mum, adored by her kids, but she often feels that with so many pressures on her time, she doesn't give them as much as she ought to. Dinner time is an opportunity to sit down and chat together about the day, to listen to each other and relax. At the moment, Kerry is so focused on feeding them and sorting out tomorrow's clothes that she is denying herself the time with them and of course the nutrition she herself needs.

Cure factor: Get the kids to help her with the food preparation. It's time they can enjoy together. Make sure she cooks a balanced, healthy meal that they will all eat, then sit down, relax and eat it together. No more eating up the leftovers while doing the dishes.

Late evening: After the children are sorted and settled, Kerry needs to give some more attention to herself and her own wellbeing. As she starts to benefit from the results of Hibernation Diet living, she'll find that she isn't feeling exhausted at this time of day, so she'll feel able to start doing some resistance exercises at around 8.30 in the evening, then she should spend around 20 minutes on these. At first perhaps twice a week, then gradually building up more repetitions and a third session as she finds herself feeling more energetic.

An hour before going to bed:
By this time, Kerry's liver will have used up its resources, so she needs to feed it up. She can take her honey in one of the drinks suggested on p.38, or if she prefers, just on a piece of bread or toast or a couple of crispbreads.

Overnight recovery: Kerry's current eating pattern just hasn't given her body a chance to do the overnight recovery work. With these changes, she will start to see the benefits very rapidly. Her skin and hair will improve, she'll feel brighter in the morning, the tiredness and irritability will be a thing of the past, and she will also sleep much better. And while she's doing all that, she'll be shifting that excess weight too, especially as she steps up the resistance work.

So What *Am* I Eating?

You know what you're eating, don't you? But it might be worth a closer look at the major food groups.

FATS

Saturated fats, or 'bad fats' come from anything that is animal fat. That might be a burger, fat-rich bacon, butter, full-fat milk, the delicious crisp skin on roast chicken, potatoes roasted in lard, the traditional English breakfast, and every takeaway you buy, whether it's Chinese, Indian, Italian or a fish supper. In the average British diet, these 'bad fats' can account for something like half our daily calorie intake. Fat intake should be less than 15 per cent and that should be coming mainly from non-saturated fats.

Non-saturated fats are found in vegetable sources like olive, sunflower, sesame, flax and pumpkin oils and oily fish. These kinds of fats aren't stored as fat but instead get used by the brain and other vital organs. We need these kinds of fats for good skin, joint flexibility, blood circulation and mental concentration, both as adults and children, but only in small amounts. The best sources are salmon, herring and mackerel. So read the nutritional labels carefully in the supermarket.

PROTEINS

The building blocks of life, they're often called, and they are vital not just for energy, but also for all the repair and maintenance work that we need our bodies to do. There's an outmoded notion that you can only get 'real' protein from meat. That isn't true at all. Veggies need not fear. In fact, protein is available from a host of sources. You just need to know where they are. Fish is an excellent source, doubly so because fish is low fat and includes essential Omega 3 oils, so fish is a great pillar in the Hibernation Diet. If you don't eat fish, you can look to lean meats like organic free range chicken (no skin), lean lamb, beef or pork. For the veggies, beans are an especially rich protein source and carry almost no fat. They're also good GI reducers because the protein, fibre and low-fat content absorb glucose into the circulation without sudden peaks. Soya is immensely protein-rich and also contains important phyto-oestrogens, natural plant hormones, especially important in the female menstrual cycle and menopause.

Linseeds – not the same as linseed oil – also contain these wonderful plant hormones.

Dairy products like cheese, milk and yoghurt are also good protein sources but watch out for fat content. Cheese, especially, can be very high. Low-fat alternatives still contain the protein, so look to those to keep the fat levels down.

Different people respond in different ways to what they eat

Take a look at two sisters, Sylvia and Maria, who eat the same quantities of carbohydrates in their diet, but they do it in different ways.

Sylvia gets her glucose from within a balanced mix of low GI foods like wholegrain breads, rice and pasta, plus she eats a lot of fruit and vegetables.

Maria eats the same quantities of carbohydrate calories, but she gets hers from processed sugars, corn syrup, cakes, sweets, crisps, chocolate and from highly processed supermarket microwave meals.

For both, the same total amount of glucose is going in, but the output is another story.

Sylvia's balanced intake provides fructose for liver glucose storage and replenishment. It keeps her blood glucose level stable right through the 24-hour period, including while she's sleeping.

Maria, on the other hand, is regularly creating high blood glucose levels because of her concentration on refined sugars which in turn over-stimulate her insulin production, forcing her blood glucose back down with a crash.

Maria is activating her own fat production because of her eating patterns. She's making herself fat, not because she is consuming too many calories but because she is consuming the wrong kinds of calories.

She feels constantly exhausted as she shifts from glucose highs to glucose lows and back again. Her stress glands are reeling while Maria craves sweet foods. Her response sees her reaching out again and again for a fast-food fix, setting the whole cycle in motion all over again a dozen times a day.

Her liver is still famished. It isn't getting what it needs. She's pumping in foods that it can't access to make glycogen for her brain, so she is starving in plenty. Loads of calories, an empty liver, a hungry brain and too much cortisone.

She can't concentrate, she's incredibly forgetful, and her immune system is poor so she keeps on catching every virus that's around. One moment she's almost on a high, the next she's sunk into misery. Her hormones are so muddled up, they don't know what to do, so she's also having bouts of real depression and anxiety.

So two sisters, two similar intakes if you count the calories, and two totally different outcomes.

By the way, Sylvia weighs in at a healthy 9½ stone, while Maria is over 14 stone.

CARBOHYDRATES

Be sure that you have grasped the difference between complex carbohydrates and simple ones. The complex carbs come in food like wholegrain bread, wholegrain cereal, rice and pasta. These are low GI, take your body quite a while to break down, and therefore give you a good, stable fuel resource for a long time without sudden peaks. They're also good sources of fibre. Complex carbs are also in starchy vegetables like potatoes, corn, parsnips and yams.

Simple carbohydrates in isolation are instantly absorbed and rapidly turned into fat and are of no help to your liver at all. These are present in white sugar and white bread, highly processed foods and ready meals or takeaways. Simple sources of carbohydrate should ideally all come from fruit, vegetables, fruit juices and honey.

Fruit is good for Hibernation Dieters, all fruit. Select from apples, bananas, apricots, blackberries, blueberries, cranberries, raspberries, strawberries, cherries, dates, figs, grapefruit, grapes, mango, melons, oranges, peaches, pineapples, plums, prunes, tangerines.

Vegetables provide a great range of vitamins, minerals and proteins and are rich in anti-oxidant and anti-cancer compounds, as well as other health promoting natural plant products. They are high in fibre, the non-soluble carbohydrates (roughage), which reduce our absorption of unwanted fats and cholesterol and improve transit of food through the gut. Loss of fibre from the modern diet is mainly a result of food processing and is behind a lot of our current gut problems, including some cancers. Some vegetables, such as cabbage, lettuce, parsley, peppers, celery and cucumber can be eaten raw and this is a great way of replacing some of that lost roughage since cooking reduces it dramatically.

FOOD FOR THOUGHT

At the heart of the food matter

It was only at the turn of the twentieth century that heart disease began to emerge as a real problem. For every one death from it in 1900, 80 died of the disease by 1980. Indeed, the disease was so new to medicine that it wasn't until 1925 that an article first appeared in the professional medical journal, *The Lancet*.

The kind of high animal fat, highly refined foods that had been available only to the rich then began to become available to everyone. The luxuries of preserves, sugar, sweets and far greater quantities of meat filtered through into the diets of the many rather than the few. A developing industrial economy was raising wages. People could afford more of such tempting tastes.

An agricultural economy that provided food from smallholdings started to give way to an industrial one where people moved rapidly away from the land and its healthy diet to work in cities and towns. Here, they began to search out different foods and they longed for the once unavailable luxuries that set the menu for the decades ahead and have so damaged our general health.

The food we eat is the key to the modern epidemic of cardiovascular disease.

Fortunately there is now a growing public desire to eat more healthily, and a recognition that maintaining a healthy weight isn't only about appearance and self-esteem. Heart disease is the biggest killer in the western world.

Coronary heart disease is really a breakdown of our blood-vessel function. It begins with a tear in a blood vessel, which the body repairs with a kind of band-aid composed of lipoproteins. These lipoproteins then become the focus for the build-up of more material from circulating blood and this is where cholesterol comes in. The higher the fat content of the blood the greater the build-up of these band-aid repairs, known as plaques. Cholesterol content of these plaques varies but may rise to as high as 70 per cent and cholesterol is a potent marker for potential heart disease. Eventually the plaques grow to such an extent that the blood vessel gets blocked. If it's a coronary blood vessel, the outcome is a potentially fatal loss of oxygen supply to the heart.

Nathan Pritikin, a businessman who was diagnosed with heart disease in his forties, developed a dietary regime based on low fat, low protein and a high proportion of unrefined carbohydrates. He increased his exercise level and amazed his doctors by later showing no signs of his condition. He proved that where heart disease has developed it may be reversed.

When Nathan Pritikin died, a post-mortem showed his arteries were those of a young person and were plaque free.

We know that being overweight predisposes us to far greater risk of heart disease, but it's worth bearing in mind that you can be obese and fit just as easily as you can be lean and unfit. There is a whole package of other factors that enter the equation: smoking, level of exercise, psychology and attitude, genetic factors and lifestyle.

As we have become became steadily less active throughout the twentieth century, and our diet has become increasingly packed with processed, highly refined fast food with more and more artificial additives, so the rate of heart disease has increased, alongside obesity and Type 2 diabetes.

That emphasis on refined grains devoid of fructose has led to greater and greater production of adrenal hormones because we are leaving our livers without access to new fuel.

One of the reasons adrenal hormones are such bad body news is that over-production of them leads to a large quantity of fats swirling around in the bloodstream. That means a greater accumulation of these plaques, which in turn increase the risk of coronary heart disease.

On top of that, adrenaline raises blood pressure and increases heart rate, adding still more stress to the cardiovascular system.

It's well documented that deaths from stress-related heart disease rise during periods of social crisis. On an individual level, many of us will know of someone who worked in a highly stressful environment and whose heart condition has been at least partly ascribed to that.

The links between diet, lifestyle, obesity, stress and heart disease are clear for us all to see.

The Hibernation Diet targets obesity and stress by optimising recovery during Slow Wave Sleep. Its principles help to moderate the risk factors in the development of cardiovascular problems.

A diet low in saturated (animal) fats, rich in plant nutrients and with good complex carbohydrates, plus fish, lean meat, eggs and low-fat cheese protects against heart disease.

This is the crux of the Hibernation Diet. Our Diet contains all the necessary food sources and micro-nutrients (vitamins and minerals) for energy. It offers us the possibility of a life free from cardiovascular stress. Regular exercise is also vital. This should include a mixture of low-level aerobic exercise combined with short periods of resistance exercise to optimise recovery and fat burning during Slow Wave Sleep and to maintain weight control.

FEMALE FOOD

Women approaching the menopause will benefit enormously from following the Hibernation Diet. They will reduce their production of the bone-destructive cortisone and will fend off the ageing process as well. Risk of osteoporosis increases dramatically for middle-aged women, but the Hibernation Diet will dramatically cut the risk to you.

Another effect of calmer adrenal glands is that libido is not suppressed – another one of cortisone's damaging effects. Cortisone reduces production of the important sex hormones, creating an imbalance that favours stress hormones and drives the menopause forward. The Hibernation Diet's emphasis on natural fructose tilts the balance back to the right position and pulls back from the drive towards early menopause so prevalent these days.

Look especially to soya to help at this point in your life. It contains important phyto-oestrogens, natural plant hormones, and in countries with a high intake of dietary soya, women come through the menopause quite naturally and without the grief of mood swings, sexual problems, tiredness and irritability so common here in the west. Linseeds – not linseed oil – also contain these wonderful plant hormones.

For younger women, especially those who find points of their menstrual cycle impacting upon their overall mood and wellbeing, will also see major benefits including a reduction in PMT and sensations of bloating.

Our fertility is in decline. Something like one in four couples is having problems conceiving a baby, and the male sperm count has fallen by 40 per cent in the last half century.

Feeling under stress does nothing to improve your chances of conceiving. Conception rates rise when people go on holiday and escape the turmoil of their normal environment. Perhaps they eat a healthier diet when they are less rushed as well. Again, evidence that too much cortisone is to blame for fertility decline is piling up, so if you're looking to conceive, the Hibernation Diet can be a very big help.

FOOD AND CHILDREN

When TV chef and father of two, Jamie Oliver, took on the challenge of improving the quality of school dinners in London, he found that the new food had benefits beyond the straight nutritional one, which takes around three months to filter through.

Within just two weeks, there were clear changes in the behaviour of the children. Their concentration levels were better because they were eating fructose in fruit and vegetables; they were less aggressive and more interested. Some of them had never eaten these items in their lives before.

The high-fat/high-sugar/low-nutrition diet deprived their young brains of the energy required for good mental processing and acuity. Adding fructose from fruits and vegetables gave them that mental energy.

A knock-on effect would be calmer adrenals. Cortisone inhibits production of the human growth hormone (HGH) and a longer-term study would show improved growth. In situations where children are exposed to acute stress, production of growth hormone stops and they fail to grow. The connection is clear. Cortisone inhibits growth.

GIVE THE DOG A BONE

You probably know someone who has fractured a hip and perhaps had a hip replacement. The load-bearing hip is the bone structure most vulnerable to fractures as we age, for both men and women. Both sexes lose bone mass from early middle age onwards although the problem is greater for women after the menopause when they lose the protection of their hormones. Hip fractures put a significant number of people in hospital and place a huge burden on the health service. Cortisone is the bone-degrading hormone and too much of it is a big factor in osteoporosis (porous bone disease).

The Hibernation Diet gives you a good intake of natural fructose from fruit, vegetables and honey and will provide stable liver glycogen and blood glucose levels, preventing chronic over-production of cortisone. We need a lot of nutrients to maintain good bone mineral integrity. In a high saturated-fat, high sugar diet, the ones that would be deficient are calcium, magnesium, zinc, boron and vitamin C. Vitamin C is vital for the construction and maintenance of collagen, a protein, which provides bone with strength and elasticity (rather like a steel support in a concrete wall).

A LIFE ON THE OCEAN WAVE

Vitamin C deficiency used to cause scurvy among sailors who didn't have access to fresh fruit. It was quickly remedied when lemons and limes were provided on board. Now, it's a key condition of our modern propensity for processed foods which destroy the vital vitamin in their preparation. The Hibernation Diet stresses the importance of vitamin C and the need to get it from fresh sources. Our bodies can't store it, so we need to get fresh supplies.

IMMUNE FOOD

Scientists worked out over 30 years ago that refined sugars damage our immune systems. If we take in 100 grams of refined sugar, it will suppress white-cell production for several hours. White blood cells are the ones that fight off infection. Children today get up to 200 grams of refined sugars daily in the food they eat, sometimes even in one sitting. A litre of coke contains 100 grams of sugar. It's back to that fight between cortisone and fructose. The cortisone is released into the bloodstream because the liver hasn't been able to get fructose, and cortisone is the long-term suppressant of our immune systems.

High levels of fatty acids and cholesterol in the body also damage immunity, where any energy imbalance will rapidly dilute our capacity to fight off infection.

Our modern diet, with its highly refined sugars and starches and its low nutrition value, is seriously damaging our immunity and leaving us wide open to everything from Avian Flu to a steady rise in what we thought was a disease of the last century, before the dawn of antibiotics: Tuberculosis (TB).

THE JUNK FOOD JUNGLE DIET

You've already read a lot here about how junk food and good health just can't line up how over-processed and nearly nutritionless food doesn't just leave your system unable to run at anything like maximum efficiency, it also makes you mentally disabled. You suffer from poor mental processing ability; you don't latch on to things as quickly as you ought to, and your brain seems sluggish (it is).

Too much saturated fat cuts back on something called EFAs, essential fatty acids. These are vital to get the brain working properly and for the best signal transmission between your brain cells. Without these, your mental railway lines have no reliable signalling. Without discipline, you probably won't be surprised to learn that its conditions like dyslexia, dyspraxia and attention deficit disorder (ADD) and hyperactivity (ADDH) that emerge in children.

Research with children suffering one or more of this group of disorders has proved beyond doubt the importance of nutrition in managing them. Supplements of EFAs have led to dramatically improved behaviour and concentration levels.

A study of 60 school children, half of whom were given vitamin and mineral supplements, and half who were given a placebo, clearly revealed the importance: the supplements group saw a 10 per cent rise in non-verbal intelligence quotient (IQ) after eight months. Neither the placebo group nor the control group showed any improvement.

FOOD AND FORGETFULNESS

When you stop to think about it, memory is vital in all sorts of ways. We rely on it without any consciousness of caring for it. Which cupboard are the cups in? Which days does Nicky go to the gym? When is Dad's birthday? Which is the turning for the shopping mall? And at an even more basic level, it's our memory that gets us up in the morning, that reminds us to eat, drink, stand up, sit down and so on. We wouldn't go far without it, literally.

We would get lost in time and space. We couldn't function at work or have normal relationships with people. We wouldn't know when to be cautious or whom to trust. We'd become dangerously vulnerable.

Though we're not claiming to have discovered a means of completely avoiding any later life dementia, the Hibernation Diet will most certainly play an important part in helping your body to protect itself against these cruel conditions so prevalent today.

Foods associated with brain function include essential fatty acids from fish and plant sources. The fish group comprises the Omega 3 group, and wild fish rather than farmed are the best source. Tuna, mackerel, herring and salmon are all good sources.

Nuts, seeds and cold pressed oils from these are excellent sources of the Omega 6 group of essential fatty acids.

Both of these groups of fatty acids are vital for all membrane function and in the brain and nervous system they promote optimum signalling and transmission between brain cells. Beans, whole grains and unsaturated vegetable oils such as virgin olive oil and vitamin K are all important.

Green leafy vegetables also provide the essential B vitamins for energy production in brain cells and vitamin K help bones absorb calcium. Fruit and vegetables are excellent sources of the vitamins and minerals essential to optimum brain function.

GUT FOOD FEELING

Cortisone is one of the key hormones when it comes to developing gastro-intestinal problems like ulcers and irritable bowel syndrome. Again, too much of that destructive hormone around your system and the outcome can be these sorts of painful and difficult-to-manage conditions.

The Hibernation Diet lifestyle will protect you from these kinds of problems because of its emphasis on maintaining the adrenal glands and limiting production of cortisone to its necessary roles. Athletes who train too intensively are prone to gastric ulcers, related again to cortisone which directly degrades gut tissue.

Life, Love and Leisure

Leisure means different things to different people. It can be lying on a Mediterranean beach for a week and grilling gently in cancer-causing UV rays or abseiling down mountain sides swinging from an alarmingly fragile-looking rope.

Many people enjoy gym membership, running and jogging, cycling, golf, cross-country trails, swimming, hiking, camping for example.

It's to those of you who are already pretty active in some way that we'd like to talk now.

There's an awful lot of mythology and downright error creeping into the information about aerobic exercise, what a treadmill can do for you and how you burn fat as you run. There are elements of truth in the mix but so much misunderstanding has been muddled in that it's difficult to separate fantasy from reality, but let's get a few crucial facts down:

- You cannot lose weight simply by exhausting yourself on a treadmill or in other forms of aerobic, heart-pumping, breathless-making exercise. Only a tiny portion of the calories you burn will come from fat stores. Most will come from degrading your muscles.

- Aerobic exercise is excellent for improving your general health and wellbeing, for building stamina and toning muscles. It helps to lower blood pressure and improves circulation too.
- It is resistance work that will really impact upon weight loss. The repetitions and regularity of your resistance workout all add up to encouraging your body to do what nature intended it should: use your fat stores for night-time repair.
- You can treble the number of calories your body burns from fat stores at night by doing a resistance workout three times a week.
- Resistance work at these levels will not turn you into the World's Greatest Strong Man or Woman. It will not give you muscles to embarrass Arnold Schwarzenegger nor will it in any way damage your natural internal chemistry.
- What it will do is make you feel better, sexier, calmer and stronger because it discourages the release of dangerous hormones as well as giving your body access to your fat stores while you sleep.
- Aerobic exercising is fine. Don't stop it if you like it. But resistance exercise is so, so much better if you're trying to lose weight.
- Don't ever fall for the tired old myth that if you don't eat before exercising you'll lose more weight. You'll just lose more muscle.

While we're overturning some of the fat fables and fictions, let's look at Hanna's story.

HANNA'S STORY

Hanna was a fantastic young distance athlete. Her stamina

was great and she had the kind of body shape to suit her running ambitions. She was ambitious and knew she could go places.

At just 15, Hanna was already competing at international level and had her own designated coach and clinician. Visiting a new sports clinic, the clinician weighed her. Hanna was 44 kg with a body fat ratio of 11.6 per cent, equal to five kilos.

'Too high,' the clinician declared. 'Distance athletes need to have a body fat ratio of under 10 per cent. Do your training and cut your calorie intake down.'

Surprised but intimidated, Hanna did as she was told and came back a couple of months later. Her weight had dropped to 37 kg and her body fat to 11.2 per cent, equivalent to four kilos rather than five.

Hanna had shed seven kilograms of weight. just one kilo was fat. The other six were all muscle protein, the very fabric that made her the promising athlete she was.

Hanna never won another race. Not only did our 'wise' clinician ruin her career, he may very well have ruined Hanna's general health. Her menstrual cycle stopped as she struggled to lose weight and she has put herself in the very high risk category for developing osteoporosis later in life. She's already damaged her immune protection, may well find she develops fertility problems and is unable to conceive naturally, plus she has invited in a whole set of other potentially serious conditions that could well shorten her natural life.

Lots of recreational exercisers also get drawn into the myth that exercise works better if you do it on a fast without fuelling in advance. The idea is that somehow your fat reserves are being better mobilised this way. It's an alarmingly popular fallacy at gyms and playing fields. But fallacy it categorically is.

If you don't fuel correctly for your exercise with the

right carbohydrates, you will not lose so much as one extra gram of fat as a result. Not one.

Carbohydrate deficiency during exercise will never, ever result in increased loss of fat. What you are doing in this context is depleting your valuable muscles.

The reasons for the confusion are simple to sort out.

It is the intensity of your exercise programme that is key to its using up excess fat during Slow Wave Sleep. When you exercise, the proportion of fat contributing to your energy output is decided not by what you've first eaten but by how intensely you work out.

For instance, during moderate (aerobic) exercise, fat contributes around 50 per cent of the energy output. As the intensity of exercise increases, the quantity contributed by fat diminishes, so that, at maximum intensity, when your heart is beating at its fastest and you're most out of breath and sweating (anaerobic), fat makes no contribution whatsoever. So as intensity increases, the proportion of carbohydrate usage rises until at maximum anaerobic intensity, all your energy is coming from carbohydrate utilisation.

So where do our carb-deprived systems make up the deficit when we haven't eaten anything before exercising? Fat can't be converted into carbohydrate. We don't have the enzymes to carry out such a conversion.

We have to use our protein reserve, and that means our muscle protein.

Muscle proteins are degraded and carried over to the liver where they are converted into glucose to make up the deficit resulting from prior under-fuelling. And guess what, it's a really silly thing to do.

To create a single gram of glucose in the liver, 2 grams of protein must be degraded within our muscles. Because not all the amino acids in muscle protein can be transported to the liver and some are degraded and oxidised within muscle tissue, it's a wasteful and destructive process.

The yield of glucose in your liver from these amino acids is no match for the protein that's been degraded from your muscles. It is not a fair trade-off. Remember, not one gram of fat will ever be used during exercise to make up the deficit of carbohydrate during exercise.

So forget about the fat fables, fictions, falsehoods and fantasies. These four are losers. Losers of muscle, not fat. If Hanna had followed the Hibernation Diet principles, she wouldn't have suffered from consequences for which she will be paying for the rest of her – possibly shortened – life.

The Hibernation Diet fuels the liver before and during exercise so that muscle is protected. The stress on muscle comes instead from resistance work because it's when your body starts repairing itself during the recovery period that your system uses the greatest amounts of your fat stores exclusively as its energy source.

The Hibernation Diet works on a liver-fuelling strategy. Already, we have a big database of athletes at various levels who have found it works for them. More than that, they have seen clear improvements in their whole mood and psychology. Although that's easy to explain from the standpoint of a properly fuelled liver, it's more difficult to separate out that emotional system that links the unconscious mind with the 'thinking' cortex of the brain. Believe us, it's there.

EVERYTHING IS IN ORDER. LIVER IS FUELLED UP; BRAIN CAN RELAX

If you were following the Hibernation Diet plan and your body could speak, that's what it would tell you. That it can't articulate the information doesn't mean you don't get the impact of it though. Your contented and happy internal organs will have a very positive effect on your whole mindset.

Exercise uses up your liver fuel far more rapidly than when you're at rest, so the experience of athletes gives us a useful, accelerated model of what's happening to the rest of us.

For some athletes, especially the seriously competitive ones, overtraining is a danger. It reduces their ability both to train and to perform to such a degree that they often start having symptoms closely akin to clinical depression.

These symptoms include lethargy, apathy, lack of motivation, loss of interest, low self-esteem, fatigue and inability to train. With the near-overwhelming evidence linking cortisone over-production to depression that we've already explained earlier, it's very likely that the key element in this sorry state is also chronic over-production of cortisone. Few athletes have so far recognised the issue, and they don't use natural fructose to hold back cortisone.

But they will now that the Hibernation Diet is explaining it clearly.

KIRSTEN'S STORY

Kirsten , who's 23, has always been very active, taking part in school sports teams for hockey, running and swimming and going to the gym on a regular basis. She always tried to eat healthily and keep slim, giving way to the odd sweet craving for chocolate or biscuits.

'In 2001 I began working in the leisure industry as a fitness instructor. I was teaching a variety of classes in various health clubs. Some were aerobic and some resistance. I was exercising at least three or four hours a day, and I thought that would make me lose weight and would tone my muscles more.

'But it didn't. It just wasn't happening.

'A few years later, I set out on a real mission to lose weight before my summer holiday. I stepped up my training on top of teaching classes. The extra was mostly cardio-based, spending a couple of hours in the gym pounding on he treadmill, climbing the stepper and long sessions on the bike. I pushed myself to around 65–75 per cent of my maximum heart rate, convinced that would shift the extra weight.

'I didn't think much about resistance or weights, and I found no change at all in the state of my physical body after two solid months.

'When I discovered the Hibernation Diet, I was suspicious. No, shocked actually. I was told I was "over-training", was "under-eating", and not getting essential nutrients. I looked and felt tired, was pale, irritable and kept breaking out in cold sweats. I had wretched stomach pains and suffered from irritable bowel syndrome, especially following the first meal after training in the morning.

'How could I not be eating enough? I wasn't losing weight. Eating less had to mean I'd lose more weight, didn't it?

'I was told the best course of action was actually to fuel my body more so that changes could start to take place. I had to take glucose and fructose in the morning, during training and at night. I had to increase my resistance training, increase my food intake using low GI foods. I was advised to work each muscle group once a week, rather than everything together, giving time for a week's recovery when the muscle fibres would be using fat reserves for the repair.

'It all seemed, well, rather unlikely, but I followed the plan on exercise and on diet. If I wanted to change the shape of my body, I'd need to eat six small meals a day, plus the honey. For my size, two teaspoons twice a day is enough.

'At first I was struggling to eat so much food. I didn't believe I would lose weight at all. Yet within a few months, my shape was changing. My muscles were much more toned and my clothes were getting loose, though my weight stayed the same.

'As my body went through further changes, I continued to train hard and work the muscles to fatigue. The diet seemed fine to me until the first day I didn't take honey in the morning. By mid-afternoon, I felt ill, looked pale and was shaking. I pushed on with no carbs but by the second day I felt really terrible.

'I ate some dried fruit then. The difference was hard to to believe. I felt a hundred times better and I've gone on doing so while I've steadily been losing weight. I've not become tired and grumpy the way so many people on diets find themselves. I've stayed with my honey morning and night and the physical changes have got better and better.

'People have been incredibly surprised by how much weight I've lost and how brilliant I feel and look. I've lost 4 kilos in the last couple of months, but perhaps, for me, even more important is the fact that I'm now carrying a fat weight of 11.9 kg instead of 15.5 kg.

'I put it down to the Hibernation Diet combined with a tough weight/resistance workout'.

Appendix
Supplements and the Hibernation Diet

TO SUPPLEMENT OR NOT TO SUPPLEMENT?

Experts are pretty divided on this question. The medical professions tend, although this is changing, to oppose supplementing diet with extra nutrients and take the view that a balanced diet will meet all our food needs.

A quick look at the nutritional content of many modern foods makes us question that view.

Patrick Holford points out in his fine book (*The Optimum Nutrition Bible*) that wheat has 25 nutrients before it is refined. Refining removes every single one of these. Four are put back in: iron and the B vitamins, B1, B2 and B3.

In Earl Mindell's best-selling book, *The New Vitamin Bible*, the author shows clearly how you can enhance your quality of life and boost not only your energy levels but your fertility and your sex life as well when you use supplements smartly.

We are all becoming more aware of what's missing in our diet, and increasingly we're taking the view that supplements are certainly useful in certain circumstances, both for treating some conditions and for preventing others from developing.

The National Science Foundation of America issued a report a few years ago which said that 88 per cent of adult Americans believed in, and used, some form of 'alternative' medicine. As early as 1998, research reports showed that half of every US health dollar was being spent on alternatives to pharmaceutical drugs. Not only are Americans looking for alternatives, but they're prepared to pay for them because neither insurance, nor Medicare, will.

Yes, that could create the conditions for an exploitative supplements industry, but knowledge is power. Know what you want and why and you are properly equipped to purchase the right products at sensible prices.

There is clear evidence of a sea change in attitudes to using nutritional and other health supplements rather than powerful synthetic drugs, which so often give rise to complications.

The Hibernation Diet takes the view that supplements can be used where they are well researched and provide benefits without any unacceptable side-effects.

Before taking any supplement on herb, do check with your doctor, pharmacist and supplement provider for any contra-indications.

NUTRITION IN HEALTH

We used to think that, when we visited the doctor or pharmacy, their advice would take into account our lifestyle and eating habits. But that was probably an illusion. Doctors tend to prescribe on the basis of the unhealthy symptoms they see, not on the 'whole person' although there are a few welcome exceptions.

Nutrition, the basis of all biology, is not taught in depth in medical school, nor in fact to most of the other professions involved in health care, bar those who make a specialism of dietetics.

Supplementing our diet with safe and natural products is surely worth careful consideration.

Food molecules, far from being simply the material that we consume at mealtimes, are the switches that activate all our biology, that activate and deactivate all the metabolic enzyme systems and pathways which characterise our biology and metabolic life.

Cells need energy. Without it, they commit a kind of hara-kiri. If not enough energy is available, the cells will sacrifice themselves. It's a siege strategy that allows remaining energy to be used more efficiently by the surviving cells. Our entire bodies behave in the same pattern. If there isn't enough energy, then we will pay a heavy price in terms of our own health.

We've seen a raft of toxic medicines being questioned and often withdrawn from use during the twentieth century. There was Thalidomide in the 1950s which led to often terrible deformities in babies of the time. We had chloral hydrate, the bromides, barbiturates, benzodiazepines, amphetamines – including slimming tablets – and a variety of tranquillisers, hypnotics, anti-depressants and other mind-altering drugs. The latest group, the SSRIs like Prozac and Seroxat, are coming under increasing scrutiny and have a backlog of legal challenges.

There are, of course, many useful synthetic and life-saving drugs, some of them genetically engineered as a result of our growing knowledge of genes. Human insulin springs to mind, and where synthetics are shown to be the medicine of choice then they should not be dismissed out of hand.

OBESITY

One cause of obesity is a diet too high in refined carbo-hydrates, sugars and saturated fats, all of which lack nutritional content. As a result, being overweight may well also mean being short of certain vital nutrients.

A daily **multivitamin and mineral supplement** would protect against any such deficiency, though it is not a cure for poor eating habits.

Processed and refined foods are almost entirely fibre free, leading to loss of muscle tone in the gastrointestinal tract. Where the diet lacks fibre a fibre supplement such as Psyllium husks may be a good idea, either in a granulated form or in capsules.

5-hydroxytryptophan (5-HTP) is a natural form of serotonin. It is available in tablet form from natural health stores. Raising levels of serotonin has been shown to reduce appetite because it reduces the amount of cortisone we produce. Cortisone makes us hungry, so lowering its production will return us to knowing when we've eaten enough to feel satisfied'.

Chromium improves insulin metabolism and so helps overweight people for whom insulin resistance and Type 2 diabetes are a high risk. Chromium is often offered in weight-loss regimes.

L-Carnitine is an amino acid and a vital part of the system that allows our bodies to burn fat and use it for energy. It's a useful and safe supplement to use during a weight-loss regime.

Garcinia Cambogia is an Indian herb. Animal studies suggest that it may be useful in weight loss regimes. No human studies seem to have been done so far. Anecdotal evidence does strongly suggest that it can help.

Agnus Castus is a herb that stimulates the recovery gland (the pituitary) and, if taken at night before bed with honey, will energise the entire overnight process of rebuilding and maintenance. Although no studies in weight loss have been done with this herb, there is strong anecdotal evidence that it can help. *Agnus Castus* stimulates production of certain hormones which in turn have an effect on the production of your sex hormones. If you are taking any kind of prescribed hormone treatment, avoid this herb.

Brancos, which are branch-chain amino acids, have been shown to be a helpful addition as part of a weight-loss regime.

Medium-chain Triglycerides (MCTs) are short-chain fatty acids which the body is unable to store. By adding MCTs as a supplement, we can speed up our normal metabolic rate by anything up to 50 per cent, which can help to increase weight loss.

Co-enzyme Q10 Overweight people often seem to have low levels of Co-enzyme Q10, an enzyme that helps our bodies to create energy out of the food we eat. Supplements have been shown in research to help promote weight loss.

Glucomamman is a natural bulking agent that has been shown to improve weight loss when taken before breakfast and the main evening meal. It helps with the digestive flow.

Green Tea Extract, containing equal amounts of caffeine and EGCG (epigallocatechin gallate), seems to increase the speed at which we use up energy, perhaps by increasing our metabolic rate. It has been used as a successful supplement in weight loss.

DIABETES

No one with diabetes, Type 1 or Type 2, should start taking alternative health medication without first discussing it with the appropriate consultant/diabetes care professional, and should never be tempted to reduce or cut out prescribed medication.

Chromium is part of the Glucose Tolerance Factor (GTF) and has been shown to improve insulin sensitivity in both Type 1 and Type 2 diabetes.

Linolenic acid needs to be converted from Gamma Linolenic Acid (GLA) before the body can use it and diabetics can have difficulty making that conversion. Supplementing with Evening Primrose Oil can help and has also been shown to improve diabetic neuropathy (degeneration of nerve tissue), a long-term complication of the condition which can lead to loss of sensation, especially in the hands and feet.

Vitamin C is especially significant for diabetics. It competes with glucose in cell uptake because both need insulin to get inside the tissues. A shortage of it leads to localised scurvy in the cells of blood vessels. Vitamin C is also vital in the manufacture of collagen, which provides blood vessels with strength and elasticity. Diabetics are particularly vulnerable to breakdown and degeneration of blood-vessel function, a major risk factor for heart disease. Vitamin C also protects against damage to circulating proteins, and against the accumulation of sorbitol which can clog up vulnerable cells such as red blood cells, nerve cells and the retina. All diabetics should consider supplementing with extra vitamin C.

Vitamin B6 is often at low levels among diabetics and has been used successfully in the treatment of diabetic neuropathy.

Biotin is of interest to diabetics because, like fructose, it seems to liberate the glucokinase enzyme in liver cells, so pulling more glucose into the liver and reducing blood glucose levels for Type 2 diabetics.

Magnesium supplements are worth thinking about. A shortage of it increases the risk of heart disease, and diabetics are already at a high-risk level of cardio problems. Research shows that diabetics tend to have low levels of magnesium.

Vitamin E (Tocopheryl) improves insulin metabolism. Low Vitamin E status increases the risk of Type 2 diabetes.

Alpha-lipoic Acid, a powerful anti-oxidant, may be useful in the prevention of diabetic neuropathy.

L-Carnitine, an amino acid, has been shown to recover some of the nerve damage in diabetics.

Co-enzyme Q10 is another potent anti-oxidant that is low in Type 2 diabetics. Supplementing with Co-enzyme Q10 produced a drop in blood sugar levels in a case study of diabetic patients.

THE IMMUNE FUNCTION

Weston Price, an American dentist from Pennsylvania, visited several countries in the 1920s in his research into dental health, which is closely linked to immune function.

He found populations in South America, Asia, Africa and the less developed areas of Europe to have much the best teeth. Why? Because the traditional diet they consumed helped to build strong immunity. In more sophisticated, westernised society, our diet concentrates on highly refined foods, including sweets, jams, sugar, white flour and chocolate. Teeth told – and continue to tell – their own tale of decline.

In the west of Scotland, Price found two distinct groups. First, on the islands were those who had excellent dental health and who stuck to the traditional diet of oatmeal, vegetables from the croft and protein from a rich variety of marine sources. Second was the group who had access to mainland foods. The mainlanders diet of refined foods brought dental health problems and saw young people making regular trips to have decaying teeth removed.

Tuberculosis found easy prey among these already weakened people. They were helpless against the virulent infection because their immune systems were already compromised by poor diet. Whole communities, once renowned for their strength and vigour, were mown down by the disease.

The study, old though it is, shows clearly the impact of sound nutrition based upon traditional, organically grown produce compared to the processed, refined and treated food of today's supermarket shelves. While hardy older generations could withstand killer bacteria, younger people were without the immune resources to put up a fight.

The addition of vitamin and mineral supplements will at least help to build better immunity. Alongside the Hibernation Diet food plan, the result will give us a much stronger capacity to fight off infection.

Fats and your immunity

The link between lowered immune function and obesity is cortisone driven. If we are releasing too much cortisone, then liver glycogen will be low. A diet high in saturated fat and refined sugars pushes the liver towards storing fat (Syndrome X) instead of converting sugars into glycogen.

As a result, we'll have a liver chronically short of brain fuel and chronically pumping out more adrenal hormones in search of it. That presence of cortisone in too high amounts undermines our immunity.

Vitamins and your immunity

Vitamins A and E are powerful stimulants to immune function.

Beta-carotene is a natural supplement with a positive effect on immune function.

Vitamin C It was the scientist, Linus Pauling, twice winner of the Nobel Prize, who was first to review the beneficial effects of adding vitamin C to our diet. Pauling saw the links between health and nutrition and noticed how vitamin C intake had declined since the time of our hunter-gatherer forebears.

Glutamine, an essential amino acid, is key in the immune system. When the body is under stress glutamine is lost and this, along with over-production of cortisone, dramatically lowers immune function. Supplementing with glutamine has proved beneficial.

Zinc deficiency lowers immune function and supplementing with it has been shown to reverse this effect.

Selenium is a mineral vital for human health. The European continent is low geologically in selenium with the result that most of the population is deficient in it. Selenium is necessary for the thyroid gland hormones, and the lack of it in our diet is contributing to the large number of people suffering from an under-active thyroid gland. Selenium is also required as a key part of glutathione, a powerful anti-oxidant enzyme vital for protecting vitamins, proteins and structural lipids in membranes from oxidative damage. High levels of glutathione are associated with longevity. Supplementing with selenium potently improves immune function.

Echinacea is a herb which has powerful immune-stimulating properties, especially useful if recovering from an illness.

DEPRESSION

Forcing our bodies into a state of biological stress has, unsurprisingly, an impact on our state of mind. The chronic over-production of cortisone affects the limbic system which regulates mood and appetite. Brain cells are deprived of energy and that causes depression. Prescribed anti-depressive drugs act by re-establishing cortisone receptors and therefore enhancing the negative feedback signal which in turn replenishes normal energy partition in the brain. Depression is a disease of brain energy depletion and is linked to memory loss in the limbic system. Biological stress can be the result of an illness of any type, and there are many prescription medications which have an unwelcome depressive impact. If we're short on energy and good nutrition, we'll make the problem worse and we'll inhibit our night-time recovery function.

5-HTP is perhaps the most interesting of all the natural supplements used to treat depression. It comes from an African herb called *Griffonia simplicifolia* and seems to be relatively free of side-effects. You can buy it at health food stores and online. It is probably as effective as the Selective Serotonin Reuptake Inhibitors, better known as the SSRIs, and is consistently less likely to cause unpleasant side-effects. With prescribed anti-depressants such as Fluoxetine (Prozac) and Paroxetine (Seroxat), many people endure problems with sleep, degrees of impotence and, perversely, clinical trials have shown that taking these drugs can actually double the risk of suicide. Instead of interrupting the flow of serotonin, as the SSRIs do, 5-HTP has the effect of helping the body's natural serotonin production process to increase. 5-HTP improves the quality of sleep, unlike the SSRIs which disrupt normal sleep. This, of course, is important in using the Hibernation Diet strategy overall because it is essential to enjoy high-quality Slow Wave Sleep to maximise our own recovery capacity. It's self-help of the true kind.

Omega 3 deficiency may be linked to depression. This group of essential fatty acids allows vital parts of the brain to communicate with each other. Because intake of Omega 3 is declining so rapidly in the western diet, supplements may be helpful.

L-phenylalanine is an amino acid which enhances mood in the central nervous system and improves morale in depressed people.

DLPA consists of two forms of phenylalinine (the D and the L type) and has been shown in a clinical study to have positive results in treating depression compared to a prescribed anti-depressant drug.

The B group of vitamins A deficiency in this vital group has profoundly negative effects on our central nervous system. It will lower concentration levels, dampen down your ability to think clearly, make it difficult for cells to 'talk' to each other and will make you feel downright miserable. As well as ensuring that you eat foods that provide good sources of the B group vitamins, a supplement is a safe and useful addition. Scientific research has shown a clear connection between low levels of B group vitamins and depression.

S-Adenosyl-methionine is an important amino acid, involved in making neurotransmitters, those tiny molecules that ultimately control how we think and feel and react to all life's situations. Because the presence of this unpronounceable substance raises the level of key neurotransmitters, it is significant in the treatment of depression.

St John's Wort is a herb that has been shown to improve mood in depressed patients in a number of studies. It compared well to the SSRI group of drugs, in terms of effectiveness, side effects and costs. It does have some side-effects and can interact with some prescribed drugs, so check first with your health care provider.

Ginkgo Biloba, a plant known to improve circulation in the brain also lifts mood in depressed patients. *Ginkgo Biloba* is potent and must be checked against other medication and herbs for interactions and side-effects. Check with your pharmacist or other health care professional.

IRRITABLE BOWEL SYNDROME (IBS)

The Hibernation Diet puts IBS right at the centre when it comes to those stress-related disorders that are driven by over-production of cortisone. Again, IBS is a direct result of our over-processed and refined western diet, something that has been proved – if proof were needed – in the massive increase of reported cases over recent years.

When we're under stress, blood is withdrawn from the gut and shunted elsewhere to contracting muscles and other tissues. This leads to a localised oxygen and energy shortage. The gut is closed down and its function reduced. If the stress continues, and perhaps is a nearly constant state, then the gut is placed in this cycle of activation/deactivation which upsets the normal balance and can lead to gastrointestinal ulceration and IBS.

The distressing symptoms are alternating constipation and diarrhoea as the gut desperately attempts evacuation, combined with episodes of swelling, wind and discomfort.

That diet of highly refined carbohydrates, sugars and saturated fats leaves the liver glycogen store depleted, which in turn pushes the adrenal glands into producing loads of cortisone, is a diet promoting IBS.

Helpful supplements may include fibre-containing products such as Psyllium, which are bulk forming and improve muscle tone, and herbs which have gut-calming potential such as ginger. peppermint, fennel, caraway, slippery elm and chamomile.

Wholegrain rice, breads and pasta are good sources of fibre and increasing these in the diet will almost certainly help IBS sufferers.

THE THINKING FUNCTION

It's an unfortunate truth of the ageing process that our memory processing gets poorer. We don't concentrate so well, and what scientists call our 'cognitive function' – our overall ability to process information using our senses – begins to slow down.

There are a number of reasons behind this. Our brain circulation can slow down as our arteries begin to deteriorate, transporting blood around less efficiently. We lose energy from our nerve tissues and the neurotransmitters that convey the signals are less efficient.

Too much cortisone in our systems is definitely a contributor to all these problems. Maybe the Hibernation Diet can't offer you eternal youth, but we can certainly and dramatically slow down the ageing process.

Here are some of the supplements that can help keep your thinking on top form.

Acetyl-L-Carnitine, an amino acid which, is directly involved in energy pathways, has been shown to improve cognition.

The B group vitamins are directly involved in all our thinking functions and a deficiency of these vitamins is implicated in a series of central nervous system disorders.

Ginkgo Biloba helps the blood flow to the brain. Studies have shown this plant to be of benefit in dementia patients. Check with your pharmacist or health care provider for drug interactions or side effects with Ginkgo.

Phosphatidylserine improves memory and cognition. It's a fat that is a critical factor in brain cell transmission and signalling systems.

CARDIOVASCULAR HEALTH AND HIGH BLOOD PRESSURE

Magnesium is vitally important in cardiovascular health. This mineral works in the energy pathways of all cells and especially in heart cells. A low magnesium level is directly implicated in poor cardiovascular function. This is thought to account (apart from other dietary factors) for the high level of cardiovascular problems in countries such as Scotland where the 'soft' water is low in magnesium.

Co-enzyme Q10 has proved to be of benefit for patients suffering from heart conditions. It raises the energy levels in heart muscle.

Carnitine is an amino acid directly involved in transporting fats into mitochondria (the energy producing units in cells) and has proven benefits for heart patients.

Glossary of Terms

Adrenal glands

These are little hat-shaped glands that sit one above each kidney.

The adrenals are essential to life and the hormones they produce, adrenaline and cortisone, are vital in human biology.

But where the adrenals produce too much of these hormones, the result is Cushing's Disease. This condition causes a variety of problems including obesity, osteoporosis, muscle degeneration, Type 2 diabetes, infertility, gastric ulcers, loss of immune function, memory loss and depression.

These are the very conditions that are so prominent among the general population. Why? Our diet and lifestyle is creating for many of us a set of symptoms that are a direct result of our over-productive adrenal glands. That over-production of hormones leads to our liver being inadequately fuelled, which in turn exacerbates these symptoms and withholds our night-time recovery mechanism. It's the correction of this unhealthy imbalance that is the purpose of the Hibernation Diet.

Adrenaline

Adrenaline, like cortisone, is one of a group of hormones known by the tongue-twisting name, the catecholamines. Others include noradrenaline and dopamine.

Adrenaline is released during 'fight or flight' episodes to raise blood glucose. It increases blood pressure and heart rate, makes you breathe more quickly and helps make short work of converting glycogen to glucose so that you have the energy to run or to fight.

But just like all the cortisoids, too much of it has negative effects. Too much adrenaline causes sweats, shaking, tremors and stress for your heart and blood-circulation systems.

If we don't maintain a healthy blood glucose supply to the brain from the liver, then these adrenal glands will release the hormones needed to go and hijack it out of our muscles, and that, as we've said before, is very damaging to us.

Bone

Bone, along with skeletal muscle, is in the fuel silo to feed that hungry brain when the liver isn't adequately supplied. The adrenal hormones are happy to go and destroy it to meet the urgent starvation from above. It's literally unthinkable that we should be left without enough energy to flee if there were a sabre-toothed tiger pursuing. Our bodies simply have to be ready and able to cope with the unexpected, and we must have sufficient energy reserves available for that eventuality. If it's between the health and quality of your bones and the need to run from the tiger, it's the last demand that'll be the bigger one. During that kind of fight or flight, energy must be rapidly released from everywhere possible and turned into a form used by contracting muscles. That conversion needs magnesium. It's bone that provides the extra magnesium and calcium required.

Brain

The *Concise Oxford Medical Dictionary* states that the brain is the 'enlarged and highly developed mass of nervous tissue that forms the upper end of the central nervous system...'

The brain has many divisions, regions, areas, glands. It is an unimaginable, vast territory housing trillions of cells and it has an infinite capacity for linking these cells electrically. We don't, though, have much idea how it manages to convert these electrical signals into functions like thought, speech or movement. It remains the least understood and most vital organ we have.

There are alternative ways of classifying the brain. In the Hibernation Diet we divide the brain into two sections: The MindBrain and the BodyBrain.

The MindBrain is the thinking part; the 'we' part. This is the higher-level functioning part of the brain, known as the cortex.

The BodyBrain is the lower part of the brain, often referred to as the limbic system. This section 'thinks' as well but we are not usually aware of it. It gets on with its job without consulting the cortex.

We think our conscious MindBrain is in full control, but that's not the whole story. Yes, we can command ourselves to speak, lift an arm, run, but only within certain limitations.

If we try to break through those limits, the BodyBrain will soon take over. You can see this in situations such as when an endurance athlete runs a race without fuelling up the liver. Blood glucose falls rapidly and the brain, stoking up its boiler, will already have activated the adrenal hormones in preparation for what it sees coming.

They'll be working flat out to degrade muscle to make more liver glucose, but it won't be fast enough for the BodyBrain which is more than likely to say 'Halt!' End of race for that athlete who didn't prepare him or herself properly for a long and demanding run.

It doesn't matter how much that athlete would like to keep running, Gold Medal firmly in mind, the ever-alert hypothalamus knows the liver is empty, knows that muscle degradation by adrenal hormones isn't getting fuel to the liver fast enough and that blood glucose is about to fall catastrophically. The BodyBrain demands: 'Throw the coma switch now!'

The athlete's high-energy consciousness is switched off. He or she will just have to lie down and wait until either someone brings new fuel or the muscle degradation and conversion to glucose manage to generate enough for a return to consciousness. The BodyBrain is in charge here.

Because it also regulates our emotional response to activity, the BodyBrain plays a crucial role in the Hibernation Diet. With the liver fully optimised and able to promote fat loss during Slow Wave Sleep, this is where the Hibernation Diet exerts its key benefits. The three regions of the limbic system which feature in the Hibernation Diet are the pituitary gland, the hypothalamus and the hippocampus.

Cholesterol

Cholesterol is a fat produced in the liver and also found in eggs, meat and cheese. It is essential to humans, used as structural material in cells, and as the material for manufacturing essential hormones and vitamin D. High levels of cholesterol are associated with heart disease.

Cortex

The cortex is the highest part of the human brain, immediately below the skull, that part associated with 'thinking'. The lower part of the brain, the limbic system, also 'thinks' but most of its thinking is done without our being aware of it. We think of the cortex as the MindBrain because we associate it with our decision-making and voluntary action.

Cortisone

Cortisone – in the United States, it's known as cortisol – is actually a group of cortisone type (corticosteroid) hormones such as hydrocortisone. You may also sometimes hear them called glucocorticoid hormones because they are so key in regulating our blood glucose level.

These cortisoids have powerful anti-inflammatory properties, and pharmaceutical versions are used to suppress painful inflammation. They also suppress our ability to attack unrecognised or aggressive cells. This is sometimes medically necessary – in the treatment of auto-immune diseases for example.

Used sparingly, cortisoids have a valuable role in treatment of various problems.

Cortisone is a 'fight or flight' hormone, so it is released when we feel under threat so as to make sure we've got enough blood glucose to meet the energy demand. It closes down the non-essential parts of the body and lets us either attack the enemy or get away very, very quickly. Too much of these hormones pulsing around and they begin to degrade parts of our bodies: parts of the system that they've closed down.

Don't go away with the idea that cortisone is all bad. It has an important positive function in protecting brain function and in treating inflammation disorders. But remember that it degrades your muscles to get at those glucose stores so as to give the liver fuel for the brain. If you fuel your brain properly, it won't need to and you can avoid over-production.

We call cortisone an 'adrenocide' only when we're describing its chronic over-production.

Without the adrenal glands and production of cortisone, humans would die, and a condition known as Addison's Disease where the adrenals do not function (President Kennedy was a sufferer) is life threatening if these hormones are not provided medically.

Enzymes

Enzymes are proteins which act as the machine tools of the body. For instance the liver contains an enzyme known as fructokinase which enables this organ to take in fructose. Other enzymes convert this fructose to glucose and still other enzymes convert the glucose to glycogen, the storage form.

Fructane Index (FI)

This index (FI) is unique to the Hibernation Diet and stems from the Fructose Paradox. Fructose is taken up by the liver for conversion to glucose and liver glycogen and at the same time it also optimises glucose uptake by its action on glucokinase (the liver glucose enzyme). In the Hibernation Diet we include foods within the Fructane Index which do not contain fructose but do inhibit rapid absorption of glucose from the gut. In this way, they reduce the GI drive of carbohydrate foods to raise blood glucose and promote insulin production. Fructose-containing foods are fruits, berries, honey and vegetables. The non-fructose containing FI foods include proteins (eggs, meat, cheese), fats (both saturated and unsaturated), beans, legumes and pulses and carbohydrates with high fibre content.

Fructose Paradox (FP)

This concept is fundamental and specific to the theory underpinning the Hibernation Diet. Fructose enters the liver from the portal vein and is converted to glucose and glycogen. At the same time fructose liberates the glucose enzyme and this allows the uptake of glucose into the liver for conversion to liver glycogen. Thus liver glycogen capacity is optimised, blood glucose stabilised and the brain provided with the fuel it needs. In essence, the core of the Hibernation Diet. It is found, combined with glucose, in honey.

Gluckinese – the glucose enzyme

This enzyme is found in the liver and is responsible for the entry of glucose into the liver after a meal. In the Hibernation Diet we classify glucokinase as the laziest enzyme in the human body. It spends most of its life locked away in the nucleus of the cell and will only act if liberated by fructose. Fructose allows for increased glucose uptake into the liver, for storage, or release if required, when blood glucose is low and the brain is short of energy. This amazing regulation of glucose by fructose we characterise as the Fructose Paradox.

Glucagon

Glucagon is smart but confusing. It's a hormone that opposes the action of insulin and raises blood glucose concentration.

In the Hibernation Diet glucagon is characterised as the hormone behind the dawn effect: that unpleasant early morning nausea, caused by not topping up your liver glycogen store before going to bed. As your blood glucose level falls overnight, your body starts to push out adrenaline, cortisone and glucagon to raise it again. It works, but glucagon leaves you feeling very nauseous.

Glucagon has another task. It blunts the speed at which protein-based foods add glucose to your blood stream. As the proteins stimulate insulin release, your body will also release glucagon to keep control on the insulin. It's for this reason that proteins appear on the Fructane Index rather than the Glycaemic Index.

Glucose Paradox

If the liver is presented with glucose, it has a problem because the glucose enzyme (glucokinase) is locked inside the cell nucleus and not available until liberated for glucose uptake. This is where our diet generally is so wrong. Its high levels of refined carbohydrates and absence of fructose leave our poor livers desperately struggling to get the glucose enzyme out so that it can convert the glucose to glycogen. The liver has to have fructose to liberate the glucose enzyme and allow it to take in glucose.

Glycogen

Glycogen is the storable form of glucose. It is found in your muscles and in your liver which then uses it to feed the hungry brain. It is the shortage of glycogen in your liver that causes us so many problems and which the Hibernation Diet approach tackles effectively.

Glycaemic Index (GI)

The glycaemic index is a measure of how quickly carbohydrate foods allow glucose to appear in the circulation. High glycaemic index foods, such as refined foods, flood the blood with too much glucose, causing over-production of insulin and a rapid fall in the glucose concentration. This rapid fall (hypoglycaemia) causes release of adrenal stress hormones with all the problems they cause.

Growth hormone

Human Growth Hormone (HGH) is hot on multi-tasking. It stimulates body growth, in particular bones and tendons and is released during exercise when it increases blood glucose concentration. Its main task, though, is in promoting recovery biology during Slow Wave Sleep. It's at that time that we produce the greatest quantity of HGH.

You may hear it called 'a fat burning hormone', though that's not strictly correct. The biology of recovery takes place because our fat reserves are used for fuel to provide energy in the highly calorie-demanding processes of repairing and rebuilding our bodies.

HGH is a key player in the Hibernation Diet because our bodies are happy to give up fat reserves in favour of repair and maintenance biology. We need HGH to make it possible, but it will only do so if the liver has been fuelled up before sleep.

Hippocampus

This part of the BodyBrain is concerned with memory and sensory mapping of the environment in time and space – so we know what's night and day; where we are relative to the bathroom, the school, the shops. This region is an important reference point for Hibernation Dieters because it contains the highest number of cortisone receptors in the brain and registers chronic over-production of this hormone with loss of those cortisone receptors as well as loss of cells.

Stress shrinks the hippocampus and those exposed to acute and chronic stress lose memory as a direct result of this 'hippocampal shrinkage'. The region has also been linked to depression, which some scientists suggest may be a direct result of stress and hippocampal shrinkage.

Hypothalamus

The hypothalamus is next door to the pituitary gland in the BodyBrain and acts as its regulator. It manages thirst, hunger, reproduction, eating, drinking, fighting, fleeing, sleeping and so on. These basic biological functions are largely outside our conscious control, and it is for this reason that we term the limbic system the BodyBrain in the Hibernation Diet.

The hypothalamus senses the intake of food and fuel and if there is a deficit in liver-fuel intake (as in a diet high in sugars and fats) the hypothalamus will inform the pituitary, which will then activate the adrenal hormones to look for some liver food.

Insulin

Insulin is a hormone, which is why Type 1 diabetics who are lacking it can't take it by mouth. The stomach enzymes just destroy it before it gets to the bloodstream.

Insulin moderates our blood glucose level. When we eat, the pancreas which contains the insulin-producing Islets of Langerhans move into action, releasing enough insulin to lower the blood glucose to a healthy level.

If blood glucose rises too rapidly – from too highly refined and glucose-laden food or drink perhaps – then the pancreas can overproduce insulin, causing the blood glucose to crash dangerously. Too low a level of glucose in the blood is a far more immediate danger than a slightly elevated one and can mean its victim being just minutes away from a coma or at real risk of injuring him or herself if he's working with machinery or driving a car. It's these kinds of peaks and troughs that the Hibernation Diet sets out to avoid.

Hyperinsulinism can be the outcome when we eat too much refined carbohydrate and sugar. The liver ends up converting its sugars into fats instead of glycogen. The result? A chronic shortage of glycogen, which in turn makes the adrenals pump out cortisoids in a desperate effort to correct the problem. Cortisone, by the way, makes us hungry, so off we go and eat again, hence the link between cortisone and obesity. This condition and the over-production of cortisone causes insulin resistance and Type 2 diabetes.

Exercise (including resistance exercise) improves insulin sensitivity so it helps to fend off obesity and Type 2 diabetes.

Insulin-like growth factor

This group of hormones is released by the liver, in tissues and from muscle. Their production is stimulated by Human Growth Hormone, released during Slow Wave Sleep to promote recovery. They are released in pulses throughout the 24-hour cycle but the most important time is during recovery sleep.

There are two groups known as IGF1 and IGF2.

Leptin

Leptin is a hormone released from fat (adipose) tissue when these fat stores are full. This hormone reduces the impulse to eat and increases energy expenditure. It comes from something called the 'Ob gene' and if this gene is missing, obesity results. But most obesity is associated with leptin resistance when the hormone is produced in excess but the signal for reduction in eating is not heard. It's our old friend, cortisone, that leads to leptin resistance.

Limbic system

The limbic system is the lower part of the brain which overseas and regulates all the metabolic processes required to keep us alive, heart and circulation, breathing, digestion, eating, reproduction and so on. It is also the part of the brain involved in emotional response. Known as the BodyBrain in the Hibernation Diet.

Liver

A generous and kindly organ, your liver. Most of what it does is for the benefit of other organs and tissues. The functions include detoxification, glucose metabolism and the processing, storage and distribution of foods and energy.

It is the liver's store of glucose as glycogen that keeps the brain supplied. Without it, the brain can't survive and packs off the adrenal hormones to search for muscle to degrade and convert to glycogen – fast! Without that fuel, blood glucose falls dangerously and rapidly, starving the brain and leading rapidly to unconsciousness.

The liver is the central organ of the Hibernation Diet. Its relatively small-sized fuel store creates challenges that need to be managed through smart eating.

The modern western diet, rich in saturated fats, refined

carbohydrates and sugars, results in chronic liver depletion and this in turn leads to obesity, heart disease and Type 2 diabetes, osteoporosis, infertility, memory loss and depression via adrenal hormone over-production.

That's what the Hibernation Diet is changing.

Luteinising Hormone (LH)

Luteinising hormone is a key recovery hormone. It promotes testosterone production in both men and women and testosterone is a muscle-building hormone, stimulating repair and rebuilding during recovery.

Muscle

There are three types of muscle in the human body: cardiac or heart muscle, the smooth muscle which runs the lungs and digestion, and the skeletal muscle.

Skeletal muscle is important in the Hibernation Diet because this is the tissue (along with bone) which is preferentially degraded if the liver is not fuelled optimally. It's the fuel silo that the adrenal hormones chase in search of brain food.

Neuropeptide Y (NPY)

We could call it the Hamburger and Chips Hormone (HCH) because this hormone is the one that sends us rushing off to the takeaway. Its release is stimulated by cortisone on the war mission to find glucose for the liver, so it features as one of the bad guys in the Hibernation Diet. This hormone really forms the link between our body's screaming that it's under stress and our overeating because we're flooded by adrenal hormones. In other words, what the Hibernation Diet is setting out to change.

Pituitary gland (Recovery gland)

The pituitary gland is part of the limbic system or BodyBrain, and has a crucial part to play in the Hibernation Diet.

This gland is a big, big player in the Hibernation Diet.

We know it as the recovery gland because it orchestrates the production of all the recovery hormones during Slow Wave Sleep, so taking care of this gland at bedtime is critical.

The pituitary is a schizophrenic gland. On the one hand it produces recovery hormones. On the other, it's the power behind these adrenocides, these dangerous adrenal hormones like cortisone and adrenaline that are so very damaging in large amounts. The pituitary has two switches: one for adrenal hormone production and the other for recovery hormone production.

Because, as we've already seen, our diet is failing to fuel up our liver adequately, the adrenal pituitary switch ends up in a permanently 'on' position.

What the Hibernation Diet does is to re-establish the balance in favour of the on' switch for recovery hormone production.

Slow Wave Sleep

Slow Wave Sleep is the crucial part of our sleeping pattern. It is normally the first four hours of sleep that are the deepest, and our brain waves then register a very deep and slow pattern. This is the time when our recovery biology is at its optimun level. It's when we are repairing, maintaining and reconstructing new tissue. This period of sleep mobilises and burns fat stores exclusively, providing the calories for all that rebuilding work.

Statins

Statins are a group of drugs that inhibit the production of cholesterol.

Testosterone

Testosterone is a male sex hormone and also a tissue-building (anabolic) hormone. It is released during Slow Wave Sleep. Like all recovery hormones testosterone does its work at the expense of fat. Testosterone is one of a group of hormones known as androgens secreted from the testes.

Thyroid gland

The thyroid gland, located in the neck, regulates metabolic rate and calcium metabolism by releasing three important hormones: thyroxine, triiodothyronine and calcitonin.

Although the thyroid is critical to controlling metabolic rate it is not included in the Hibernation Diet because the two conditions associated with thyroid malfunction – hypothyroidism and hyperthyroidism – both require medical intervention. Any attempt to lower or raise the production of these hormones should be done under the supervision of a doctor.

Bibliography

Peter G Bursztyn, **Physiology for Sports People**,
(Manchester University Press, 1990)
> An excellent popular book on exercise physiology which
> demolishes the myth comprehensively that aerobic burns fat in
> any significant quantity.

Mark Nathan Cohen, **Health and the Rise of Civilisation**
(Yale University Press, New Haven, 1989)
> Shows how the change from hunter-gatherer lifestyle to farming
> has had dire nutritional consequences for us.

Patrick Holford, **The Optimum Nutrition Bible**
(Piatkus, London, 1997)
> Excellent introduction to the relationship between nutrition and
> health, drawing on studies from the last few decades.

Joseph Katz and J. Denis McGarry, **The Glucose Paradox:
Perspectives**
(*J. Clin, Invest*. The American Society for Clinical
investigation, Vol 74, December 1984) pp.1901–9.
> Shows that glucose is not taken up by the liver in normal
> circumstances without fructose and that the western diet, high in
> refined carbohydrates and sugars, will not lead to formation of
> liver glycogen.

Joseph LeDoux, **The Emotional Brain**
(Phoenix Division of Orion books Ltd, London 1998)

> Explains the limbic system which connects the thinking brain
> (cortex or MindBrain) via the limbic (BodyBrain) with the body.

Paul Martin, **The Sickening Mind**
(Flamingo, London, 1997)

> Explains how mental states are linked to biology via the limbic
> system and how the mind can impact upon physical health. Paul
> Martin's book shows that mental states and physical states are
> interconnected by bridges in the limbic system.

Earl Mindell, **The New Vitamin Bible**
(Souvenir Press, London 2005)

> This is the ideal reference guide to finding your way around the
> multitude of vitamins and supplements that are available now.

Caroline M. Pond, **The Fats of Life**
(Cambridge University Press)

> A clear and easy-to-read account of just what fats are, where we
> get them and why they are essential to life.

Weston A. Price, **Health and Physical Degeneration**
(DDS Keats Publishing Inc., New Caanan, Connecticut
1939)

> Weston Price was one of the early pioneers who showed the link
> between diet and physical decline when communities changed
> from traditional foods to modern processed foods. The change was
> immediate and dramatic and within one generation the decline in
> dental, physical and biological health had become obvious.

Anson Rabinbach, **The Human Motor**
(University of California Press) Berkeley, 1990)

> Shows the relationship between mental and physical fatigue and
> the nineteenth-century interest in the balance. It's a relationship
> that has been largely ignored in the twentieth century but is now
> making a comeback through the Hibernation Diet.

Maisie Steven, **The Good Scots Diet**
(Argyll Publishing, Glendaruel Argy 1985)

Maisie Steven, an expert on dietetics and nutrition, explains how eighteenth-century rural Scots were renowned for their health and vigour and how this was lost in the nineteenth when they flooded into the central lowland cities to provide labour for the industrial revolution.

About the Authors

Mike McInnes is a pharmacist who founded ISO Active with his wife, Theresa, and his son, Stuart, in 1997. ISO Active specialises in a nutritional approach to health and exercise. Mike has spent ten years researching and refining his knowledge of liver biology and function as the foundation for the Hibernation Diet.

Stuart McInnes is the founder of the Edinburgh Festival of Sport Science, and has researched the liver fuelling strategy for appetite control.

Maggie Stanfield is a freelance writer and editor, who lives and works in Edinburgh, and runs her own agency, www.writtenwords.co.uk.

ISO Active have developed their liver fuelling strategy through work with many athletes in different sports and this research led to the dramatic conclusion that the body could burn fat during sleep if it was fuelled before going to bed. This resulted in the development of the weight loss plan known as the Hibernation Diet.

ISO Active recommend a number of products to use in this diet:

Hibernation Honey for use at night
Honey Stinger bars and gels as liver fuelling snacks
ISO Torque +, an exercise fuel for use during training or competition

For further information please contact:

ISO Active Ltd   ISO Active Ltd
57–59 South Clerk Street   46 Queen Street
Edinburgh   Glasgow
EH8 9PP   G1 3DS

0131 622 5101   0141 847 0565

Or visit www.isoactive.com or www.hibernationdiet.com